REMAKING THE BODY

Rehabilitation and change

Wendy Seymour

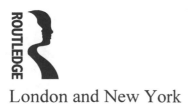

London and New York

First published in 1998 by Routledge
11 New Fetter Lane, London EC4P 4EE

Simultaneously published in the USA and Canada
by Routledge
29 West 35th Street, New York, NY 10001

Typeset in Sabon by DOCUPRO, Sydney, Australia
Printed and bound by KHL Printing Company (Pte) Ltd, Singapore

British Library Cataloguing in Publication Data
A catalogue record for this book is available from the British Library

Library of Congress Cataloging in Publication Data
A catalogue record for this book has been requested

ISBN 0-415-18601-3 (hbk)
ISBN 0-415-18602-1 (pbk)

REMAKING THE BODY

Foreword

The human body has become a dominant theme of both popular and commercial culture in Western societies over the last decade. The cultural thematisation of the body in contemporary society is a consequence of a variety of social changes and movements, including the women's movement, gay liberation, technical changes in medical science, and commercial changes in the use of the body as an icon of contemporary consumerism. These multiple social changes have focused commercial activity on the human body as a measure of aesthetic excellence; thus there is endless popular discussion of thinness as the fundamental criterion of female beauty, athleticism as the final mark of masculinity, and physical power as a necessary component of political authority. In our culture, looking good has become the equivalent of being good.

It is not surprising that many contemporary sociologists have contributed to the emergence of a new sociology of the body, analysing the contemporary self as a reflexive identity in popular culture. The contemporary self is a narrative structure within which self-reflexivity is conducted around a series of stories within the individual life-cycle. These biographies of the self are increasingly integrated into a set of projects within which the body becomes an inseparable and necessary component of modern identity. The cultivation of body image is the principal mechanism for the presentation of self in modern society and, therefore, our culture has become highly narcissistic. This development explains the explosion in physical education, dietary regimes, slimming manuals, vegetarian cookbooks and athletic equipment.

The new emphasis on physical image of the body as a sign of

the self can be regarded as the final stages of a profound secularisation of Western culture which had its origins in the seventeenth century, particularly in Descartes' revolutionary proclamation, 'I think, therefore I am'. It was this slogan that launched the great modern project of individualism, materialism in science and the mind/body dichotomy. One could argue that in late modernity the Cartesian dualism of mind and body has been overthrown by a secular commercial culture that celebrates and elaborates the body as the great modern symbol of self-authenticity. In this respect culture is a repeat or restatement of a seventeenth-century baroque culture that celebrated the importance of the body to sensibility and religiosity as a counter attack to the Puritanical negation of the body and regulation of sexuality. The Puritans knew well that the regulation of the soul required a government of the body, and this converged around the notion of diet as the government of both spiritual and physical existence. In our society, however, diet has become the platform and basis for enhanced sexuality and pleasure, a complete reversal of much of the discourse and practice of conventional Puritanical culture.

Modern consumer society invites us to celebrate the possibilities of pleasure derived from a cultivated and enhanced embodiment. The principal challenge to this comes from aging, death and disability. It has been often argued that contemporary culture, with its emphasis on youth and beauty, has shunned, precluded and negated the fact of death. Death has become medicalised, excluded from everyday life, and denied through the representation of the eternally youthful body brought about by the modern funeral industry. A similar argument might also apply to aging and disability, which are increasingly regulated, medicalised and controlled by legal regimes. The new conception of aging, for example, emphasises the importance of activity theory; earlier theories such as disengagement theory are abandoned, and the importance of continuous involvement in leisure activities for the elderly is emphasised. Despite this, as the population of Western society ages, there is an increasing ratio of dependency on the employed population, a marked increase in degenerative disease and hence a growing burden on the welfare system.

It is within the context of these corporeal challenges (death, aging and disability) that we should appreciate the significant achievements of Wendy Seymour's penetrating and comprehensive study of the life-world of people with a disability. On the surface this is a book about various forms of paralysis associated with spinal cord injury. The people in this book are victims of massive physical injury resulting from accidents, or the victims of muscular dystrophy and cerebral palsy. Remaking the Body must, however, be read at a much deeper level. It is a profound study of the 'ontological insecurity' of human beings when faced by constant danger, uncertainty and risk in areas where the great contingencies of life constantly bear in upon us. *Remaking the Body* can be read therefore as a moral sociology of embodiment that explores the themes of ethics and embodiment in a medical context. It could also be read as a contribution to the endless human discussion of theodicy which in its Christian context is an exploration of divine mercy in the face of human suffering and misery.

But this is not a pessimistic study. Indeed, it is a moving account of the everyday experiences of men and women attempting to rebuild and reconstitute their lives against overwhelming odds and with a remarkable degree of human vitality and courage. Wendy Seymour's book presents a brilliant account of the remaking of human bodies in post-traumatic contexts where, through individual stoicism and collective support, men and women are able to rebuild and rediscover a new self. To use the language of Anthony Giddens, it is a study of the prospect of a 'second chance', that is, the prospect of rebuilding and reconstituting life after a profoundly damaging catastrophe. In this respect, *Remaking the Body* is also a contribution to the neglected area of existential sociology, namely a moral analysis of the nature of self-identity and personal continuity in a world that threatens us constantly with meaninglessness and disabling anomie.

The book, however, moves beyond an account of people with a disability as merely victims of circumstance and society to look at the ways in which the process of reconstructing and reconstituting the self also involves people in a process of reconstructing society. People with a disability are the subjects of profound authority and regulation, where disability is produced by endless medical discourses, by everyday medical institutions and by the routines of medical inspection. The person with a disability is in the literal sense a 'fiction' of medical constructions. Wendy Seymour's study of spinal injury victims is also an account of their subtle resistance to the normalisation of disability through medical practice. These men and women have been embraced by medical institutions which, through various processes of rehabilitation, retraining and relocation, attempt to convert them into 'normal subjects'. From the point of view of medical practice, the body is an object, a substance upon which medical practices are performed. The body under the medical gaze is an object that has the same status as the chairs and tables that occupy domestic space. Within the clinic, bodies are the focus of medical inquiry, experiment and treatment but they are also the objects of social policy, social work routines, political debate and religious reflection and manipulation. From the point of view of the reflexive subject, however, mind and body cannot be separated. Who I am depends upon a unique and peculiar form of embodiment, *my* body in this place at this time. Wendy Seymour's book is an attempt to provide an account of life from within subjective existence and personal embodiment. It is a reflection on emotions from the point of view of the damaged body. Her study is also an account of the struggle people with a disability encounter in expressing themselves through sport, sexual activity, cultural practices and social relationships.

Remaking the Body is an intelligent contribution to the development of the sociology of the body, bringing together profound theoretical insights into the nature of human identity and demonstrating the value and importance of qualitative data in the analysis of human lives. It contributes to a philosophical discussion on the nature of the human body, achieved through a sensitive study of injury. One can speculate that Wendy Seymour in fact examines the distortions in modern social structure via an analysis of the tension in the human torso. The body here becomes an enduring metaphor of the disorders of the social body. *Remaking the Body* is therefore, in my view, a contribution to ethics via an analysis of embodiment. In this respect, it points us towards Spinoza, whose view of philosophy was based upon a new model of the body which asserted that 'we do not know what the body can do'. For Spinoza the body far surpasses the knowledge we have of it, just as thought surpasses the consciousness we have of it. For Spinoza the new model of the body does not imply any devaluation of thought but, more importantly, a devaluation of consciousness in relation to thought. Therefore a discovery of the unconscious is as profound as the discovery of the unknown quality of the body. *Remaking the Body* is not only an extension of sociological knowledge but a profoundly moving contribution to our understanding of what the body can do.

PROFESSOR BRYAN S. TURNER
DEAN, FACULTY OF ARTS
DEAKIN UNIVERSITY
AUGUST 1997

Contents

Acknowledgments

A cknowledging the many people who have influenced this book is a daunting task. Foremost I am indebted to the twenty-four people whose experiences form the substance of this study. I am extremely grateful for the knowledge they have entrusted to me, and mindful that I must not repay my informants' generosity by increasing their vulnerability.

Three small internal research grants from the University of South Australia enabled me to undertake the research upon which the book is based. The quality of the book has been greatly improved by the meticulous help of Penelope Griffin in revising the final manuscript, and the excellent formatting ability of Liz Preston. I appreciate the generous assistance of librarians Sandy Gray and Don Di Matteo: Sandy in the early part of the project and Don more recently. I have been most fortunate in the support that I have received from Bryan Turner. While the excellence of his scholarship is irrefutable and his own output prodigious, his generous support of my work has been critical to its evolution and to its completion.

The role of the people I have named above is clear, but a project such as this involves the contributions of other people whose influence may extend further back in time. I have drawn on the rich, insightful data given to me by the informants in order to interrogate key questions in sociological theory. They have opened up their lives for my inspection. It seems churlish, if not methodologically reprehensible, if the writer does not also reveal some aspects of her own life that may have influenced the work.

Although it is not of the same dramatic nature as the disabilities experienced by the men and women in this study, I have had a progressive arthritic condition involving joint pain and restricted movement since adolescence. While the disability may have legitimated my right to conduct the research in the eyes of the informants, it may also have influenced the information I sought, and the importance I attached to aspects of the material. It has certainly influenced my life in ways that bear on my current work. An earlier career as a health professional was cut short by the destructive disease-process in my body. Well-versed in biomedical views of the body, I was led by subsequent studies in anthropology to return to a medical domain—a spinal injuries unit—to conduct field research, and to begin what has become a compelling quest to explore the body. While no closer to reaching an answer, the search has revealed amazing insights into the strength and resilience of the body, into the impermanence of categorical thought, and into the fluidity and creativity of human embodiment.

Many more people have supported me in this longer journey. Though I have not named these people specifically, I know them, and I acknowledge their contribution to my life.

Finally, the generous spirit and unconditional support of Peter Whittam have fortified me throughout the process, as have the love and understanding of my daughters Jo and Kate.

Introduction

The men and women who have provided material for this research have experienced profound and permanent body paralysis. Extensive body paralysis represents a serious assault on the embodied self because a damaged body disrupts the self. This study explores the impact of major physical impairment on embodiment, and the processes involved in re-embodiment after catastrophic injury or disease. 'Embodiment' always indicates, following Merleau-Ponty (1962), that perception is from a vantage point, namely the body. A 'self' cannot be a disembodied agent. *Remaking the Body* examines how people reconstitute their embodied self after major personal disaster. The word 'body' in this book is used interchangeably with the word 'embodiment'.

The public discourse of disability focuses on individuals who achieve success in endeavours that are valued in the able-bodied world. The extraordinary nature of the achievement is implicitly contrasted with the tragedy and loss that most people with damaged bodies must endure. The sporting achievements of paralysed men, for example, correlate with dominant values associated with male bodies, and yet these achievements do not threaten the status quo. While this study will explore the important construction of a 'body for others', its focus is directed to the more fragile, private and intimate concerns, often obscured in public discourse, that are involved in the construction of the 'body for self'. This book addresses intimate issues, but it is not revisiting the restrictive construction of the private tragedy of disability. While the bodily betrayals (Featherstone & Hepworth 1991), leakages and unpredictabilities involved in these conditions disrupt intimacy, the reconstitution of intimacy must inevitably engage with the damaged body. A person needs a body, and (some) body, in order to be intimate. The damaged body is interwoven with social expectations in the active process of self-reconstruction, because the body for self and the body for others are both part of the on-going work of re-embodiment.

'Personal tragedy theory' (Oliver 1990, p. 10) has underpinned thinking about disability, but powerful critiques of this theory have come from social scientists such as Albrecht (1992), Murphy (1987), Oliver (1990) and Zola (1981). They perceive disability from a particular vantage point, namely a damaged body. Despite social science criticism, the individualised locus of bodily loss and the medicalisation of the 'problem' continue to reinforce and enhance the diversionary power of this discourse (Oliver 1990, p. 6).

In exploring the processes involved in remaking the damaged body, this book must also address the issue of rehabilitation. The inevitability of formal rehabilitation in a medicalised context, and the subsequent need to defer to formal agencies for services, invest these bodily changes with the labels and expectations of the rehabilitation industry. However, this exploration confines itself neither to the reified concept of disability constructed by the 'disability business' (Albrecht 1992, p. 27), nor to the parameters of bodily restoration defined by the rehabilitation industry and its commodified services (Albrecht 1992, p. 28). Indeed this book attempts to divert attention from the 'special' life of a person with a disability and the sequestered world of rehabilitation to suggest that the processes involved in remaking the body are precisely the same processes in which we all engage throughout our daily lives in constructing the embodied self. If reflexivity is forced on us all in the modern world (Giddens 1991), then body care and body work are necessary practices of everyday life. Eating, exercise, washing, grooming and dressing, for example, are activities in which the body engages in routine tasks of bodily management. Such practices are, in effect, everyday rehabilitation. Making, unmaking and remaking our embodiment are on-going activities.

As embodied social agents, our lives are preoccupied with the production and reproduction of bodies. Although the people in this study have been forced to confront their embodied selves, their experiences are vivid examples of the very processes in which we all engage. The fragmented bodies in this study highlight the continuous, largely taken-for-granted work involved in our embodiment. Although the word 'rehabilitation' has been appropriated by medicine and the rehabilitation industry, the concept of rehabilitation employed in this study relates to broader issues of embodiment which may take place in contexts far removed from the agencies and auspices of conventional rehabilitation. The book is about remaking the body, not about formal rehabilitation.

The book engages a series of theoretical, methodological and analytical themes. In its focus on embodiment, the research is situated within the general theoretical approach of the sociology of the body. In recent years social constructionist approaches have dominated this sociological field. While providing useful accounts of the power of social discourse to produce the body, this perspective also obscures the body. While radical constructionists would claim that the body is no more and no less than discourse, this study focuses on the crucial role of embodiment in the reconstitution of self. In this respect, the analysis draws upon the phenomenology of the body that has been developed by Merleau-Ponty (1962). Moves to reconcile and integrate the dichotomous positions represent a vigorous and lively debate within sociology. The purpose of the book is to test the integration of the dual approaches in sociological theory by careful interrogation of empirical data. In identifying the problems associated with these positions, the study will contribute to a more integrated and incorporative theory of embodiment.

Four analytical strands, each relating to a key component of the analysis, shape the argument. The first strand relates to the frailty and vulnerability of the human body, characteristics that are epitomised by the bodies of the informants in this study (Scarry 1985). The second strand addresses the context in which the reconstitution occurs. Re-embodiment takes place in a context of crisis, danger, fear, uncertainty and risk. Although damaged bodies represent these characteristics in vivid form, they merely highlight the features that constitute the context of 'high modernity' (Giddens 1991), namely contingency, uncertainty and risk. The third strand projects into the future. In utilising the theme of second chance derived from Giddens (1991, ch. 1), the quest for new opportunities and possibilities motivates the active engagement in the project of self. Powerful narratives may confine vulnerable bodies to the narrow parameters of an established rehabilitative product and deflect attention from other more expansive bodies. This fourth strand addresses the institutional and social impediments that underlie the reflexive project.

Chapter 1 identifies recent developments in the theory of the body which provide the framework of this book, and acknowledges the specific analytical themes that inform the research. A description of the characteristics of the people and the conditions that constitute the field of study is followed by a discussion of the methodology employed in the construction of the data and the subsequent analysis and writing of the material into a formal study. The research material is the substance of chapters 2, 3, 4, 5 and 6. The body is situated in a social context and is subject to its categories. It is through these social categories that the body is revealed in both a phenomenological and a social sense. Thus the processes involved in remaking the body are explored through the discussion of issues relating to appearance, relationships, sport, sexuality and bodily continence, key contexts for bodily activities. The interview data are often couched in terms of conventional masculine and feminine categories since these understandings underpin the informants' views of their bodies, and their aspirations for re-embodiment. For many of the informants, body disruption represents an opportunity, often the first opportunity, to confront the gendered nature of their embodiment, and in some respects, to change it. The last chapter, chapter 7, summarises key aspects of the argument and identifies critical issues for the future. Rapid development of technology in recent years presents a spectre of hitherto unimaginable possibilities for the body and for social theory more generally. Remaking the body takes on radical meaning in the new millennium. The last pages of the book will foreshadow exciting areas for future investigation.

Although the sociology of the body is an important development within sociology, this rapidly expanding area still lacks a coherent research framework for addressing 'the body in society and society in the body' (Turner 1994, p. x), the objectivity of the body as well as its 'corporeality or bodiliness' (Turner 1994, p. xii). Damaged bodies, fractured identities, disrupted social relationships, crisis, danger, risk, loss, change, opportunity, intimacy and embarrassment are recurrent themes throughout this book. The nesting of theoretical, empirical and analytical dimensions within each other in the study constructs a coherent context for the exploration of embodiment in conditions of crisis and uncertainty. An earlier work established my commitment to the exploration of damaged bodies (Seymour 1989); *Remaking the Body* reaffirms and extends this analysis. In exploring the experiences of people who live in and with damaged bodies, this study contributes to the understanding of embodiment in a context of competing demands in a rapidly changing world. In remaking their bodies these men and women are also remaking their world.

1 The body

'It is as clear as the nose on my face.' 'He knows as much about me as I know about myself.' 'She knows me like I know the back of my hand.' 'It is as obvious as I stand before you.' These phrases are commonplace and seem uncontentious. But is the body obvious? Can we be so certain about our noses or the backs of our hands? We possess our bodies more intimately than we can ever possess any other object, but does intimacy guarantee knowledge? Is it possible to know our own bodies, let alone the bodies of others?

In our quest to know the body we seek help from others. We delegate the task of knowing the body to people we consider to be experts. We turn to others to find out about our own most intimate possession, our own bodies. A doctor may probe the body to see if a cancer is lurking within its dark interior spaces or to check if the valves of the heart are functioning appropriately. Can we be sure of the doctor's interpretation of the examination? Will doctors tell us what they find? What view of the body underpins the investigation, guides the interpretation of evidence and directs subsequent practice? We rely on experts, but there are many body experts, and many contradictory views about the body. Is it possible to know the body? Can another know more about my body than I know myself? What is a body? Is there a body to know?

Such intriguing questions have provoked the minds of a wide variety of scholars throughout history. Andreas Vesalius recorded the complexities of the interior of the body in his anatomical drawings of dissected cadavers. Michelangelo's sculptures, drawings and paintings captured particular qualities and characteristics of the human

1

body. The meticulous work of Renaissance artists depicted the body in a naturalistic manner, rather than iconographically, and added new knowledge of the surfaces and interiors of the body to the emerging scientific understanding of the body (Davis & George 1993, p. 131). The rise of science challenged traditional and theological ways of viewing the body. New scientific understanding depended on experience and experiment to justify propositions rather than on revelation or faith (Davis & George 1993, p. 130).

The body was penetrated in order to understand its internal processes as well as its structure and form. Descartes (1596–1650) and La Mettrie (1709–51) secularised the body by comparing it to a machine, claiming that since it was a set of physical properties in motion, the body could be explained by the laws of physics (Davis & George 1993, p. 131). Similarly, Paracelsus (1493–1541) suggested that the body could be seen as a set of chemical reactions explicable by the laws of substances (Davis & George 1993, p. 131). Harvey's studies of the circulatory system (1578–1657) employed a systemic analogy to examine the action of a particular organ in relation to the function that it performed for the maintenance of the organism (Davis & George 1993, p. 131).

This legacy assured the development of biomedicine and its practices. A relentless search for more accurate ways to measure bodily functions, developments in asepsis and anaesthesia, and continually refined technologies for viewing parts and functions of the body have greatly enhanced interventions into the body. The normal, routine body that was thus created responded to the laws of physics and chemistry. The search for the cause of illness or disease focused on symptoms demonstrated by sick individuals. The work of Pasteur, Lister, Koch and Virchow in the nineteenth century investigated the cause of illness at a cellular and micro-organismic level (Davis & George 1993, p. 156). This work, the basis of the germ theory of illness causation, proved to be extremely influential in the rise of medicine. By demonstrating the mechanism of disease causation, and subsequently by locating the specific cause of a particular disease— the doctrine of specific aetiology—medicine was able to move out of the empirical world of observation and classification characteristic of the dissecting room and clinical practice into the laboratory, where it became established as a science of universal bodily processes (Davis & George 1993, p. 157).

Illness was located in the individual body; it resulted from natural events acting on universal bodily processes. The body was seen as predictable, measurable, universal and constant: a collection of moving parts and processes which could be fixed by medical intervention if they faltered. The positivism of medicine conceals the connection between scientific knowledge and social and intellectual interests (Short 1994, p. 227), yet medical knowledge is as much a social product as it is a product of the natural sciences (White 1994, p. 216).

Science provided new and secular definitions of the world which justified the existing social and sexual division of labour (Doyal 1979, p. 147; Laqueur 1990, p. 108; Martin 1987; Oakley 1986, p. 10; Schiebinger 1987, pp. 42–83; Shilling 1993, ch. 3). While the positivism of medicine has been remarkably successful as the basis for the establishment of the profession, this perspective has been most detrimental in its influence on our perception of men's and women's bodies. If the body is a natural phenomenon, then it follows that men's bodies and women's bodies are natural entities. The association of biology with nature confirms the 'naturalness' of particular bodies for men and particular bodies for women. The differences between the bodies of men and women—and the superiority of men's bodies—is established by these dichotomous categories. The opposition of male and female bodies inherent in biomedical thought establishes the basis of inequality between men and women in other areas of social life. Articulated within the paradigm of science and legitimated by the power of medicine, the naturalness of these categories is seen as unproblematic. 'It's only natural' that women rear children, 'it's just commonsense' that men should pursue careers because that is 'just the way things are', are typical of the biological bed-rock that is used to justify enormously complex structures of discrimination.

THE BODY IN SOCIOLOGY

The development of sociology as a discipline is characterised by disinterest in, or at best ambivalence toward, the body. The preoccupation of classical sociology with urban and industrial society (Turner 1991, p. 6), the maleness of the founding fathers (Shilling 1993, p. 26) and the privileging of abstract theorising distanced sociology from the taint of biologism, and in the process, from the body itself. Apart from some work of the symbolic interactionists, notably the work of Erving Goffman (1959; 1963; 1967), sociology has evolved until recently with very little, if any, concern for embodiment.

Biomedicine has been a fertile field for sociological study. Over the last forty years the practice, paradigm and profession of medicine have occupied many social scientists, and scholarly enterprises have developed around each of these areas. The works of Talcott Parsons (1951), Eliot Friedson (1963; 1970a; 1970b; 1976), Fred Davis (1963), Julius Roth (1963), Anselm Strauss and Barney Glaser (1975; 1980), and Erving Goffman (1968) have been particularly influential in this respect. However, while these studies opened the medical domain to scrutiny, most importantly by highlighting the client's perspective of medical processes, they did not challenge the positivist basis of medical knowledge. The medical view of the body remained a self-evident fact. These studies focused on the manner clients dealt with this phenomenon and with the institutions and professional workers involved in their care. The body itself eluded sociological interest.

Yet it is extraordinary that embodiment has remained peripheral to sociology for so long. Embodiment is our life-long obsession. Eating, sleeping, washing, grooming, stimulating and entertaining our bodies dominate our lives. Our bodies preoccupy and delight us. Despite interest in 'life issues' such as birth, maturation, death and deterioration, and the social importance of 'life events' such as socialisation, marriage, divorce and burial, the integral role of the lived body in these events has been neglected within the social sciences. Since we all have bodies, a focus on human embodiment would provide a compelling opportunity for communication and shared experience (Shilling 1993, p. 23).

More recently, the theme of the body has been employed in the work of a number of scholars. Writers have engaged the body in a variety of ways which fit with their particular ontological positions and epistemological concerns. While the body seems fundamental, the body variously appears and disappears in the works of different scholars. From obdurate fact to ghostly discourse, from embodied actor to a body-less body: a range of approaches to the body can be demonstrated within the discipline of sociology. Substantial sightings of the body can be seen in the works of Berger and Luckman (1966), Bourdieu (1978; 1984), Connell (1983; 1987), Elias (1978), Foucault (1979; 1981), Frank (1991b), Giddens (1990; 1991), Goffman (1963; 1964), Merleau-Ponty (1962), Shilling (1993), Turner (1984) and others, although many of these perspectives may appear contradictory. Despite the variety of positions expressed by these scholars, Turner suggests that the body has always existed as an undercurrent within social theory, that there has always been a 'secret history of the body' (1991, p. 12; 1992, p. 31). Although mainstream sociology has ignored the embodied agent, it nevertheless presumes a notion of embodiment. This opacity has created serious problems for the development of sociological theory.

Recent interest in the body

Despite Turner's claims of a continuous, covert history of the body, the recent animation of the body as a lively topic of analysis within sociology can be attributed to a number of significant factors.

Postmodernism has elevated the body as a key theme in contemporary activities as well as in scholarly thought. New technical possibilities and cultural changes have brought into question former legal and medical boundaries of the body. Questions of desire, sexuality and transgression have moved into the centre of the sociological stage (Turner 1991, p. 18). The role of pleasure, in particular the immediacy of feeling, is an obvious site of subversion. In contemporary society the body becomes a project which is continuously produced by means of unlimited consumption of goods and services (Falk 1994); the body as performance and display takes centre stage (Shilling 1993, p. 35). Working and reworking the aesthetic body is a human obsession (Falk 1994; Featherstone 1991). The difficulties faced by sociology in relation to bodies may merely reflect the confusion and complexity of the body in society.

It is clear that issues of gender, sexuality and biology within feminist critiques of patriarchy have been influential in vitalising interest in the body within sociology (Turner 1991, p. 20; 1992, p. 45). More recently, men's studies have engaged with the slip-stream of this work and redirected the focus of inquiry to men's bodies. Although some work in this area seems dedicated to the politics of retribution, other work stands out as making a substantial contribution to a genuine sociology of the body (Connell 1987; Connell & Dowsett 1992; Hearn & Morgan 1990; Hearn 1994; Kimmel 1987). Ambiguity of current male and female sex roles may account for the developing interest in the role of the body in men's self-esteem. Body image may be one of the few remaining areas in which men can distinguish themselves from women in the face of women's increased participation in the public sphere; men can express and preserve traditional masculine roles by literally embodying them (Mishkind et al. 1987, p. 47).

Ironically medicine, a focus of earlier sociological critiques, has also played a significant role in increasing the prominence of the body in practice and in theory in recent times. Reduction in the incidence of conditions such as cardiovascular disease and cancer is associated with attention to the body, and looking healthy is an outward symbol of one's inner commitment and social responsibility (Mishkind et al. 1987, p. 46). Improvements in medicine have played a part in increasing longevity, dramatically changing the demographic shape of the population. Yet ironically, if people live longer, their bodies are subject to an increased likelihood of injury or disease (Hetzel & McMichael 1987). Medical services may be seen as victims of their own success as people live longer but with an increasingly diverse collection of chronic conditions. The economic costs of longevity have themselves heightened concern about the body (Shilling 1993, p. 34). Coupled with dramatic innovations in organ transplantation, reproductive technologies, cosmetic alterations and sexual realignments as well as concerns associated with the HIV and AIDS crisis, these issues have raised profound philosophical and ethical dilemmas about what it is to have or to be a body (Turner 1991, p. 22; 1992, p. 46). Sport has also played a role in increasing interest in the body. The perspective of the body as a machine, exemplified in medicine (Lupton 1994, p. 59), reaches its zenith in sports science. The raw material of athletes' bodies becomes *the athletes'* machines, as specific parts of the machine are isolated and transformed into effective components of competitive performance through the application of scientific knowledge (Shilling 1993, p. 37). Similarly, the electronic media and films such as *Robocop* and *Blade Runner* have unsettled our certainty about what constitutes a body, and where one body finishes and another begins. Operating at the interface of the body and technology, virtual reality muddies the boundaries of previously uncontroversial categories (Balsamo 1994; Kroker & Kroker 1988, p. 15). Even those styles of films that previously aimed to provoke our fears of people from unknown places or aliens from outer space now find that a more effective source of horror lurks within the hidden reaches of our own bodies (Shilling 1993, p. 38; Martin 1993; Kroker & Kroker 1988, p. 12).

It is clear that the influence of Foucault lies behind much recent sociological preoccupation with the body. Just as Foucault's focus on the regulation of the body and on the surveillance of populations as 'the two places around which the organisation of power over life was deployed' (Foucault 1981, p. 139) was an explanation of the urban crises of the late eighteenth and nineteenth centuries, so too can the rediscovery of the body in the late twentieth century be seen as a response to the political anxieties of our time (Turner 1991, p. 24). Foucault's concern with productive and disciplined bodies related to the needs of emerging capitalist society. At this stage of advanced capitalism our concern is not for the productive body as grist for the industrial mill, but for bodies that must present themselves in a manner that fits the needs of the consumer society (Falk 1994; Featherstone 1987). The specific sociological concern with the body in the last days of the millennium may well be a concern with the body as a limitation, as an impediment to growth and possibility (Turner 1992, p. 11), as increasing numbers of us deal with our anxieties associated with ageing, dependency, retirement, Alzheimer's disease, HIV and AIDS. Burgeoning new industries have developed sophisticated pharmaceutical, surgical, mechanical and computerised means to extend the potential of our frail, unreliable, inefficient and vulnerable bodies, yet these may prove to be offering frustrating opportunities since the body has ceased to be a predictable, stable aspect of our lives. The body is becoming a less substantial and certain phenomenon in the everyday world. In the Western world, the body has increasingly come to be seen as a project to be worked on as part of individual self-identity (Shilling 1993, p. 4). In high modernity the body is the site upon which people may choose to experiment with ideas about what constitutes a beautiful, an erotic, an efficient or a healthy body. While in the past the body was seen as a mere receptacle for the self, the body has itself become the site of multiple projects and influences in high modernity. The boundaries of the body have become permeable, permitting the reflexive project of self and externally formed abstract systems to enter (Giddens 1991, p. 218). The body has become highly reconstructable. We can be other than that which we are.

The dual approach

Approaches to the body that have arisen within the social sciences and the humanities can be categorised in two ways. Sociology can be seen to have taken a dual approach to the body (Turner 1992). While foundationalist perspectives see the body as a lived phenomenon, anti-foundationalist approaches view the body as a product of discourses about the nature of social relations. The epistemological perspectives of social constructionism and anti-constructionism relate to these ontological positions. In anti-constructionist theory the body exists independently of any form of discourse; in contrast the construction of the body through discursive practices is axiomatic to the social constructionist position. Structuralism, poststructuralism and phenomenology have provided lively contributions to recent sociological debate. In terms of these broad categories, the structuralisms relate to the category that sees the body as socially constituted through historical discourses, and phenomenology to the perspective that asserts the phenomenological nature of the lived body. In its efforts to demystify the concept of the body by deconstructing existing discourses about the body, postmodernism is most closely associated with the anti-foundationalist approach.

The work of Foucault represents the most influential social constructionist approach, but although the body is explicit in his work, the body itself is unexplicated. In terms of Foucault's epistemology the body exists only as a product of discourse; we learn more about the power embedded in discourses about the body than we learn about the body itself. Foucault was not concerned with the lived body; the body for Foucault was present as a topic of discussion but absent as a focus of investigation (Shilling 1993, p. 80).

Constructionist perspectives have profoundly challenged the dominance of biomedical understanding of the body. Positions within this perspective range from radical constructionism which claims that there is no body beyond the social discourses that construct it, to a weak or minimal constructionist position which recognises the influence of social categories on the body, but not their domination. Feminist analyses of cultural texts have illuminated powerful processes that have bound women to specific representations of femininity and alienated women from their bodies (Butler 1990; Cranny-Francis 1992; Gilbert & Taylor 1991). Although social constructionists may debate amongst themselves as to the degree of social production involved in construction of the body, all would agree that the body is significantly shaped and constrained by society.

Despite the important achievements of anti-foundationalist sociology, social constructionist analyses have themselves been subjected to considerable scrutiny. Constructionism has been accused of resting on a number of contradictory intellectual and value premises, and of failing to tackle its inherent relativism (Bury 1986). If all forms of knowledge are part of discourses, and relative to time and context, as constructionists claim, why should constructionism be different? Constructionist analyses too are based on ephemeral knowledge, contingent and haphazard views of reality, and dispensable categories (Bury 1986, p. 155). Does constructionism assume an exempt status for its own knowledge base, perspective and methodology (Bury 1986, p. 151)? The paradox that constructionism must jeopardise its own position in the process of demonstrating the cultural production of all knowledge lies at the core of the critique of this perspective.

Turner's book the *Body and Society* marked a critical point in the exhumation of the body within the discipline of sociology. Published in 1984, this work established Turner's commitment to the body in terms of understanding changes in the mode of production. However Turner attributes his affirmation of the central role of the body in understanding everyday life to more recent re-explorations of German social theory (Turner 1992, p. 3). In the writings of Weber, Heidegger, Gehlen, Heller and Habermas, Turner observed the well-established contrasts between 'the immediacy, practicality and sensuality of the life-world and the regimentation, externality and constraints of the institutional structure of the social system' (Turner 1992, p. 3). Embodiment—the lived body—is a sparse term in the English language. The German language is more particular in this respect, and commonly differentiates between the body as *Körper* and the body as *Leib*: between the objective, exterior, instrumental and institutionalised body and the subjective, animated, living, experiential body. It is this double nature of human beings that expresses the ambiguity of human embodiment (Turner 1992, p. 42). The *Leib/Körper* distinction confronts the weakness of Cartesian sociology which has treated the body as *Körper*, rather than as simultaneously *Körper* and *Leib*.

In their concern with the lived body, phenomenology and philosophical anthropology have provided significant correctives to anti-foundationalist accounts of the body. The work of Schilder (1964) and Merleau-Ponty (1962) are significant in this respect. Schilder argues strongly that *Körper* cannot be viewed in isolation from *Leib*, that the objective body must not be seen as distinct from the inner sensations of the subjective body. The body is a unity of *Körper* and *Leib*: an outside and an inside. The body is always present, not merely a product of sensations. Sensations get their meaning only from this unity, which is one of the fundamental units of our experience (Schilder 1964, p. 283, cited in Turner 1992, p. 56).

Merleau-Ponty also deferred to a distinction in the German language: that between *Umwelt*, a setting, and *Welt*, a world. He claimed that man [*sic*] has not only a setting, but also a world (Merleau-Ponty 1962, p. 87), and later, that man 'is not a psyche joined to an organism, but a movement to and fro of existence which at one time allows itself to take corporeal form and at others moves toward personal acts' (Merleau-Ponty 1962, p. 88). In establishing the grounds for integration of psyche and organism, for organic process and human behaviour, Merleau-Ponty posited a fluidity and interconnectedness between *Körper* and *Leib*, between objective and subjective body. For Merleau-Ponty, consciousness is embodied, and therefore can only be understood within the context of lived experience. Human agency and interaction involve more than just knowledgeability, intentionality and consciousness (Turner 1992, p. 35). If sociology is the interpretative understanding of social action, then embodied human beings, human personality and consciousness embodied in human material, are engaged in that action. The integration of body and mind is the starting point for a theory of embodiment.

The pro- and anti-constructionist positions at their most polarised are thus: while constructionist analyses discount the body in favour of social forces, naturalistic approaches obscure the role of social forces on the body. Constructionist perspectives cannot account for the presence of the lived body; biological perspectives fail to acknowledge the presence of society. Each perspective professes to be about the body, yet each perspective distorts the body in terms of its particular epistemological base, and neither provides a satisfactory account of the body in society. It is clear that biomedical discourse has created particular bodies, but constructionist analyses have failed to illuminate the experience of a sick body. Powerful analyses have exposed the discursive construction of gender inequality, but the phenomenology of men's and women's bodies remains hidden. Missing from each position is a commitment to embodiment, to a consciousness that is always and already embedded in the body. Implicit in the notion of embodiment is the fact that human beings are embodied social agents. Human beings do not simply have a body, they *are* bodies, and human beings are actively involved in the development of their bodies over their own life-cycle. It is only through the concept of embodiment that the body can be understood in terms of its corporeality, its sensibility and its objectivity (Turner 1994, p. xi). These polarised perspectives have hindered the growth of a robust sociology of the body, essential to the development of sociological theory more generally.

Implications of the dual positions

Anti-foundationalist sociologists have produced vigorous accounts of the influence of social discourse on the body. Illumination of the powerful forces implicated in the construction of the medicalised body, men's bodies, women's bodies, old bodies, young bodies, beautiful bodies and erotic bodies has had a profound impact on understanding the relationship between the individual and society. It is not hard to see that the explanatory success of these accounts could persuade us that there is nothing more to know about the body, that the body is no more than a product of cultural knowledge and discourse. In failing to account for the critical role of human embodiment in the constitution of social systems, these analyses provide only partial knowledges. While relegating the body to the periphery of their investigations such studies can contribute to but cannot in themselves succeed in the construction of a sociology of embodiment. The body is a corporeal phenomenon, which not only is affected by the social system but also forms a basis for and shapes social relations (Shilling 1993, p. 100).

How can the experience of pain be accommodated within a perspective in which all biological realities are fabrications? It is undeniable that the experience of pain and a person's reactions to it are to a large extent socially mediated, but pain is also experienced as an attack on the phenomenological and embodied self. The feeling of pain is generally seen as a problem of the sensory system which can be managed or alleviated by medical means; the analysis of pain is considered to be an issue that fits within the domain of psychology. The experience and the emotions associated with pain, especially chronic pain, have implications beyond a perspective of pain as a sensory problem or a psychological issue. Starting from the perspective of an embodied agent, the experience of pain takes on a new meaning as the person acts and responds to the state of being in pain. The neglect of a sociology of pain in the sociology of health and illness (Turner 1992, p. 169) represents a serious gap in the study of embodiment.

While the primacy of rationality in early sociology, and the privileging of discourse more recently, can be seen as products of the Cartesian legacy, modern sociologists could be seen to be reproducing these binary forms. Categorical allegiance to a particular position may be a mark of an immature discipline, but advocacy of a moderate position often evokes the spectre of consensus and compromise. Destabilisation of existing narratives, particularly the dichotomous nature of social thought, is central to the postmodern enterprise. Foundationalism, anti-foundationalism; phenomenology, social constructionism; body, mind—although each position represents a substantial ontological base and a particular epistemology, these positions need not be incompatible. Recognition of a phenomenological foundation of a socially constructed body would not annihilate the anti-foundationalist argument. Would it not be possible for these perspectives to reconcile their differences and recognise the wide areas for complementarity within their seemingly dichotomous positions?

Integration of the dual positions in sociology

Turner draws on the works of a wide variety of scholars to identify areas that offer the potential for synthesis. Foucault was not concerned with the body as *Leib*, and for this reason Foucault 'rejects the idea of a universal ontology and thus rejects any attempt to think about the body as a grounding for such a universalism' (Turner 1992, p. 53). Turner has suggested, however, that although it was hidden the body was nonetheless integral to Foucault's work. Merleau-Ponty, Schilder and others were more overt in their acceptance of integration between the organic and the subjective body. It is the work of Berger and Luckman (1966) and Berger (1967), however, that Turner finds most 'congenial' (Turner 1992, p. 117) in establishing a case for synthesis between foundationalism and anti-foundationalist discourse analysis. Berger combines a foundationalist ontology with a constructionist view of knowledge, a view shared by Elias in *The Symbol Theory* (1991). Critical to Berger's argument is that although culture is socially constructed, its construction is the consequence of the very peculiar and unique biological foundations of the human animal as a 'not yet determined creature' (Turner 1992, p. 118). Turner simultaneously takes a foundationalist view of the significance of the hand in the evolution of culture and society, and supports the notion that the 'hand' is a discursive construct within a classificatory paradigm that is fundamental to human society, namely the superiority of the right hand (Turner 1992, p. 118). Although basic notions of good and evil are tied up with the fact that left-handedness is a 'sinister' accomplishment, it is the 'dexterity' of the thumb that has enabled human culture to develop endless cultural complexity. The body provides the foundational potentialities upon which endless cultural practices can be erected (Turner 1992, p. 118).

The double nature of human embodiment, illuminated by the expanded meaning of the term embodiment in the German language, provides more important substantiation for the case for integration (Honneth & Joas 1988, p. 72, footnote 6). Although Cartesian sociology has treated the body as *Körper*, embodiment incorporates both *Körper* and *Leib*. Having a body, the body as constraint; and being a body, the body as capacity: both reflect the duality represented by these seemingly contrasting philosophical positions.

Turner's call for synthesis (1992) and Shilling's declaration of the necessity for bridge building (1993) encourage sociology to rally to the same cause: a reconciliation between a view of the body as a biological phenomenon and the constructionist view of the body as a social production. The life-world, everyday life, is about the production and reproduction of bodies. Access to the life-world therefore demands a vigorous sociology of the body in order to understand the routines, conditions and practices that produce and reproduce bodies in everyday life. It is the embodied actor, not simply a disembodied consciousness, that is the site of analytical attention and emancipatory promise. The body is the key to understanding society (Turner 1992, p. 4); the neglect of a phenomenology of embodiment is a 'blind spot' in the sociology of the past (Turner 1992, p. 68). The body is a phenomenological reality, yet thoroughly integrated with society and culture.

Bodily experiences are of course strongly influenced by social ideas. Pain, disorder, loss, crisis and unreliability reflect our interpretation of what a normal body does and is, and how one should properly react to these sensations. Yet despite the overwhelming influence of society, it is still the body that feels, the body that experiences events, the body that expresses its concerns. Within the context of society the body remains a vivid, lived presence. An analysis that incorporates the phenomenology of embodiment does not deny the power of social discourse in the construction of bodies, but it recognises a broader context within which the body can be known and understood.

The proposal for synthesis calls for *rapprochement* and an elimination of dichotomous positions in the interests of a universal sociology of the body. Renouncing neither position, this reconciliatory movement is based on the recognition of the body as a simultaneously social and biological phenomenon. Although seemingly a 'middle ground', this approach is no mere compromise between two opposite positions but an exciting and rigorous attempt to develop an integrated sociology of embodiment, a sociology that recognises the importance of both the body and society, as well as of the mind. Clearly some questions will require exploration by means of one element, other questions may depend on examination in terms of another. In all analyses, however, acknowledgment of the fundamental unity of the body as lived experience and the discourse of the body as objective presence will be paramount. The advantages of an overt theory of embodiment in the development of a more comprehensive, less sectarian sociology of the body are clear. Repositioning the body will introduce the possibility of interdisciplinary research between traditional enemies, the biological and the social sciences, and closer to home, it would also offer a strong analytical grounding for a number of subdisciplines within sociology such as medical sociology, sociology of gender, sociology of the emotions and the sociology of food (Turner 1992, p. 71). Although the spectre of epistemological pragmatism haunts any attempt to unsettle established positions, the integrity of the relationship between the body, the self and society remains central to the integrated project; without it, no sociology of the body can be entertained. Ironically, a sociology of embodiment may be even more critical in conditions of postmodernity where the status of the body, and indeed society itself, is under constant challenge.

Identification of the dual approaches to the body within sociology and the implications of this polarity have occupied the first half of this chapter. Moves to reconcile and integrate these dichotomous positions represent a vigorous and lively debate within sociology. It is this robust theoretical forum that is the context for this book. The intention of *Remaking the Body* is to empirically test this theoretical position. Through careful interrogation and analysis of the experiences of people who live in and with frail bodies, the study will illuminate the components of embodiment and increase the reader's understanding of the variety of perspectives relating to the body in society. While the bodies in the study are influenced by the social system in myriad ways, the bodies also participate in their own re-embodiment and in the construction of social relations more generally. The book is dedicated to the corporeality of the body and contributes to the on-going debates associated with the sociology of embodiment, in particular to a position that renounces dichotomous positions in favour of an integrated and incorporative theory of embodiment.

THE RESEARCH PROJECT

The informants

Let me introduce you to the men and women whose experiences form the substance of this study. The disabilities these people have make them conspicuous to others. I am extremely grateful for the knowledge they have entrusted to me, and mindful that I must not repay my informants' generosity by increasing their vulnerability. While this personal information is the essence of the study, every effort will be made to guarantee the confidentiality of the informants. The names I shall use are, of course, fictitious, and from time to time I shall use other means to mask the informants' identities while taking care not to obscure the critical information that they are giving me.

All of the informants have varying degrees of bodily paralysis. While all twelve men routinely use a wheelchair, only ten of the women do so. The remaining two women can walk, but with damaged gait. Although fifteen of the twenty-four informants have sustained extensive body paralysis as a result of spinal injury, the remaining nine informants also live with varying degrees of paralysis resulting from other aetiologies. Three people were born with their paralysis, two were struck down by the sudden onset of viral infections. One informant acquired his bodily damage as the result of a neoplasm, and the remaining three developed their paralysis more slowly, but no less extensively, from different types of muscle pathologies. A more detailed description of these relatively rare conditions may identify the informants. Suffice to say that the residual bodily damage experienced by these informants is broadly similar to that of the informants who have experienced spinal injuries, but many elements are common to all disabilities, illnesses and diseases regardless of the specific nature and extent.

The age at which the paralysis occurred to the men and women in this study is also extremely variable. The three women with congenital disability have, of course, never known anything else; a further three people have lived most of their lives with gradual physical deterioration. One informant developed paralysis during childhood, while two others encountered infection-induced bodily damage as young adults. The remaining fifteen informants who sustained traumatic spinal injury did so at a wide variety of ages. The nine men range from fifteen to twenty-four years old at the onset of the paralysis; the women range from seventeen to thirty-five years—a much wider age range. The average age of the men at the time of the injury was twenty, for the women the average age was twenty-five years old—an interesting but hardly significant statistic given the small numbers and the heterogeneity involved.

Of the twelve male informants, Alister, Anthony, George, Ian, James, Peter and Ron have bodily damage that amounts to quadriplegia. Bob, David, Gerald, Ken and Mark have lower body involvement of the extent usually associated with paraplegia. Bridget, Jenny, Joy, Mary, Pam, Rosemary and Sally have lower body paralysis, while Alison's and Tina's bodily involvement is more extensive. A later complication has necessitated wheelchair mobility for Robyn, who was previously able to walk by herself. Frances and Ruth are ambulant, so their disability appears less severe.

George, Ken and Peter are now in their twenties, Anthony, Bob, David, Gerald and Ron are in their thirties and Alister, Ian, James and Mark are in their forties. Bridget, Joy and Rosemary are now in their twenties, Jenny, Sally and Tina are in their thirties, Alison, Frances, Mary and Ruth are in their forties and Pam and Robyn have celebrated their 50th birthdays.

The preceding discussion has been necessary to establish the diverse nature of my informant group. While many studies require close compatibility between variables such as age, disease category, duration of the disability, age of onset and the extent of the disability, this study explicitly does not. All of the medical conditions discussed here are relatively uncommon; some are, mercifully, extremely rare. Such infrequent incidence makes conventional correlation impossible, even if such rigour were considered necessary in a study of this type. My informants have experienced a broad set of structural and physical similarities, but the experiences of each person are unique.

Spinal cord damage and its medical management

Although the spinal cord is enclosed within the bony spinal column, it is nonetheless very vulnerable. Speed and high-impact activities, especially those activities involving cars, motorbikes, contact sports or diving, may injure, or fracture, the spinal column. This in itself is of little significance. Fractures—broken bones—usually heal quickly and well. It is the location of the soft neural cord within the bony column that makes injury to this part of the body so serious. The bony vertebrae heal, the spinal cord does not.

The severity of the disability depends on the level of the lesion (Jones & Davidson 1988, pp. 105–6); the higher the level of the lesion the greater the disability, since more muscles and sensors will be affected. Quadriplegia, sometimes referred to as tetraplegia, is a partial or complete paralysis involving all four limbs and trunk, including respiratory muscles, resulting from damage to the spinal cord in the neck. Paraplegia is a partial or complete paralysis of both lower limbs and all or part of the trunk as a result of damage to the thoracic or lumbar spinal cord or to the sacral nerve roots (Bromley 1976). The residual damage will also be influenced by the extent of the original lesion. If the lesion was complete and no nerve endings remain intact, all functions of the cord below the level of the lesion will be lost. If the damage was incomplete, part of the spinal cord below the level of the lesion will retain function. The completeness of the original lesion will thus have a significant effect on the residual abilities of different people who may be injured at the same vertebral level. As if the loss of muscle power were not enough, the damage incurred by injury to the spinal cord is usually much more extensive. Deep and superficial sensation, vasomotor control, bladder and bowel control and sexual function may also be lost.

Usually the paralysed person is immobilised in an acute spinal unit immediately after the injury to allow stabilisation of the fracture (Jones & Davidson 1988). Holes may have to be drilled in the skull and tongs inserted to immobilise the body in order to stabilise a fracture in the cervical spine (Trieschmann 1980, p. 11). A tracheostomy may be needed to ensure adequate respiratory function, and an artificial respirator may be required. Catheterisation of the bladder is instituted immediately, and fluid intake is carefully recorded in order to maintain correct fluid and electrolyte balance. Intestinal and rectal function are also likely to be impaired, so food intake must also be regulated in this early period to avoid intestinal obstruction. Pressure sores, resulting from constant pressure on prominent weight-bearing parts of the horizontal body, are a constant worry. Nursing staff turn the paralysed person every two hours day and night to change the pressure on the skin in an effort to prevent these sores (Trieschmann 1980, p. 11). Physiotherapists position the person in order to prevent overstretching of undamaged muscles and to avert contractures. The person must be encouraged to cough and to expectorate mucus from the lungs, essential early activities.

Stabilisation of the vertebral fracture usually occurs in about six to twelve weeks (Illis et al. 1982, p. 187). The second stage of rehabilitation represents a transition from the dramatic life-saving procedures of the initial, acute stage to an educational process in which the person must learn the activities necessary for daily life outside the institution. During this stage, techniques of mobility and activities of daily living are taught. Learning how to change position in bed to avoid pressure sores, learning how to transfer from bed to chair and receiving instruction in using a wheelchair are major preoccupations of this phase of rehabilitation. Care of the skin, the bladder and the bowel (Jones & Davidson 1988, p. 109) must become obsessional, since neglect of these vital parts of the body can have extremely serious consequences. People with lesions lower than the level of the lowest cervical vertebrae can achieve independence in most of these activities. Men and women with lesions above this point will be heavily dependent on family, friends, personal attendants and others for the rest of their lives (Trieschmann 1980, p. 6). Sport and vocational retraining are also important facets of second stage rehabilitation, as is learning to drive a car with hand controls for those people with low-level lesions.

KEY THEMES OF THE RESEARCH

How do men and women remake themselves after experiencing permanent bodily damage? This study is constructed around four critical themes. The first of these is the issue of human frailty. It is because of the weakness of the body and its vulnerability to injury, disease and misfortune that human beings are forced to engage in work on their bodies, to work on a body project. The experience of severe, permanent paralysis is a catastrophic event, an experience that can hardly be imagined by those of us who have endured little more neural interference than a dental injection. Not surprisingly, the body project takes place in a context of crisis, danger, fear, uncertainty and risk: the second critical theme of the study. The prospect of a 'second chance', the opportunity to reconstruct aspects of oneself after a disruptive event, is the third theme of the study. Contact with rehabilitative institutions is an inevitable aspect of severe body loss. The assumptions embedded in rehabilitation, and the implication of rehabilitative narratives for the reconstitution of the self after bodily loss is the fourth theme of the study. These four major themes, interwoven throughout the study, are drawn together by the principal theme of remaking the body.

Frailty

Although the idea of human frailty is derived from Turner (1992, p. 31) through Gehlen (1988, p. 4), the damaged bodies in this study are clearly the epitome of frailty, vulnerability and dependence. The human being is vulnerable to suffering and to pain through the very fact of possessing a body. We all live with this inescapable fact; the experiences of the informants in this study demonstrate the precarious nature of our faith in our bodies and dramatically highlight the vulnerability inherent in our embodiment.

While the body is socially constructed, as this study will go on to demonstrate, the body is a phenomenological reality—a lived body—and upon this recognition rest different possibilities. Paradoxically, it is the very vulnerability of the damaged body—the body that has failed to defend itself against disease and injury—that is the principal site of optimism. The bodies in this study have, in effect, divested themselves of civilisation; they have escaped their former social shackles. Years of socialisation, regulation and civilisation are destabilised as the body escapes its careful social constitution. The body has reasserted itself over its social domination (Seymour 1989, p. 28). In their living bodies, people with disabilities may hold the key to promising new bodies freed from the restraints of old orthodoxies with their associated inequalities.

It is not surprising, though, that the people concerned experience these events, initially at least, as a catastrophe. Paralysed bodies are deeply disjunctive bodies in terms of what counts as a body in modernity. Within this context, the disabled body has been seen as a tragedy (Oliver 1990, p. 10) because of its failure to conform to the norms of the historically created biomedical body. Yet although the word 'catastrophe' refers to a 'great sudden disaster' the meaning of the word also includes a 'subversive event' (Johnston 1976, p. 122). The old stereotype of a person trapped in a lifeless body may be transformed to a perspective where it is the living body, freed from many aspects of its social incarceration, that initiates the reconstitutionary moves.

But although the opportunity to transcend aspects of their socially constructed and physically damaged bodies presents an exciting possibility for those with disabilities, the difficulties these people face in embracing change should not be underestimated. Socialisation is a formidable force, as is nostalgia for the past. Old allegiances may be more beguiling than the promise of the future. People may feel more comfortable with old constraints than with subjecting themselves to an unknown destiny. The destruction caused by an accident or the uncontrollable depredations of a virus or tumorous growth may be more easily accommodated than damage resulting from conscious choice and individual decision making. For many people with severe disability, 'the devil you know' will always be preferable to a devil that may be much less manageable.

Crisis

The men and women in this study have experienced enormous bodily crisis. For most informants, the sudden and catastrophic nature of their injuries has plunged them into a situation of uncertainty, fear, danger and risk. But like us all, these men and women are living in a world that is also characterised by uncertainty, fear, danger and risk—a world that has increasingly targeted the body as a new surveillance zone (Kroker & Kroker 1988, p. 12).

Are the flaccid, leaking and sensory-deprived bo⟨
the men and women in this study dramatic examp
we have all come to fear in the late twentieth century? Is t⟨⟩
a vivid reminder of the body deterioration and alienation we associate not only with our own ageing, but also with the ageing of the
world? Is it the spectre of incontinence, leakages, smells and spillages
associated with severely damaged bodies that engages our anxieties
and fears about the tentative nature of our own bodily continence?
Are these bodies the harbingers of the crisis that threatens us all?
The crisis within the body parallels the crisis without—in society
itself (Kroker & Kroker 1988, p. 13).

The theme of crisis is also present in the work of Mary Douglas
(1966; 1973). The symbolic connection between disease in the body
and disorder in society, between bodily order and social organisation
is the essence of her thesis. The body provides a metaphor for
coherence and disorder in a social context characterised by crisis and
deterioration. The body has become the perfect sign of a nihilistic
culture in which the body promises only its own negation (Kroker
& Kroker 1988, p. 15). Biological fundamentalism—the generation
of a panic-based 'temperance movement' to maintain the cleanliness
and safety of bodily fluids (Kroker & Kroker 1988, p. 11)—seems
our best defence against invasion of the body by the diseases of
modern civilisation, but these measures will never alleviate our
perpetual anxiety that it will be our own body that will betray us
(Lupton 1994, p. 64). Modernity has exacerbated the potential for
personal risk and social crisis which threaten to overwhelm the frail
and vulnerable body. Yet despite our fears, it is the body that has
become the centre of political and cultural activity mediating the
tensions and insecurities of modern life.

Second chance

The prospect of a second chance, as suggested by Giddens (1991),
is a recurring theme in this study. By using a particular study of
divorce and remarriage (Wallerstein & Blakeslee 1989) to illuminate
his thesis concerning the reflexivity of the self, Giddens in his work
parallels many of the issues of concern in this study. Divorce, like
paralysis, can signal a sudden change in the circumstances of one's
life. While the prospect of either catastrophe is horrifying to contemplate, in retrospect each crisis can present new directions in life
and exciting opportunities for the future which may have been
hitherto unthinkable. The juxtaposition of danger with opportunity,
of crisis with optimism, of catastrophe with change not only parallels
the issues in this particular study, but also characterises the issues
that dominate late modernity.

By means of a reflexive construction of self, the men and women in this study have worked on their bodies and on their self-identities in novel and important ways. In the process, however, these people are also reconstructing society. Although the global world of high modernity extends far beyond an individual's activities and personal affairs, it also intrudes into the core of each individual (Giddens 1991, p. 32) and influences his or her activities and concerns. As the world is drawn into the project of reflexive reconstitution of the self, it is itself transformed by the process, reaffirming the circularity of the interrelationship between the self, body and society. Though resistant and unwieldy in many ways, society changes in response to the pressure exerted upon it. Over time new forms of bodily expression replace old categories, and different possibilities take the place of old dogmas. Society is not merely a backdrop for personal life, an external environment for human action. In struggling with intimate problems, individuals help to actively reconstruct the universe of social activities around them (Giddens 1991, p. 12). Through the process of remaking ourselves we remake the world; self building is also a world-building activity. The process that is undertaken with such purpose by people in situations of crisis is a heightened form of the very same processes we engage in continually in modern life. The reflexivity of the self as an individual phenomenon is a personal expression of the balancing of opportunity and potential catastrophe undergone by all people within the broader institutions of modernity (Giddens 1991, p. 34).

Disability has given these people a chance to rethink their bodies; it has highlighted the experience of their lived body, and the actions of others toward them. Disability thus not only provoked reflection on the body, but also presented them with the opportunity to remake their bodies in different, and maybe less restrictive, ways. The main impediment to the work of reconstitution may be the power invested in biomedicine to define what bodies should be like, and the vulnerability of the recipients of its services to accepting these definitions.

Rehabilitative narratives

Rehabilitation can be seen as a major instrument of bodily rationalisation. Disguised as 'scientific' and operating under the banner of biomedicine, rehabilitation is a powerful agent in the ratification of particular types of bodies. The 'stakeholders' (Albrecht 1992, p. 95) in rehabilitation are many, and each approaches the project from a different position and with a different goal in mind. Common to most rehabilitation work, however, is a set of moral ideas about what bodies should be like (Seymour 1989, ch. 10).

The gendered basis of biomedical thought is concentrated within this context. The 'total institutional' nature of the rehabilitative context, the vulnerability of damaged bodies, and the power of rehabilitation workers in such situations (Seymour 1989, ch. 6) enhance the gendered nature of medical practice within this specialised area. The already gendered bodies of people who become paralysed may be reaffirmed, if not substantially strengthened, by their rehabilitative experience.

Just as social constructionist sociologists have, in effect, eliminated the body in their opposition to biological perceptions of the body, rehabilitationists may also be seen to eliminate the body in their practices. This may seem surprising as rehabilitation, like medicine, has a strong commitment to the body as the object of intervention. But it is the preferencing of certain kinds of bodies, and the imperative to fit people back into society—both strongly articulated within this practice—that effectively eliminate the body. Just as the body in fully developed social constructionist argument can be seen as a fabrication of particular interests, so too can the rehabilitated body be seen as a fabrication of the imperatives embedded in a particular form of rehabilitation. The body itself disappears as powerful forces mould and shape it in particular ways.

Are rehabilitation workers unwittingly encouraging their clients to deny the lived reality of their bodies? Are paralysed people trained to manage their bodies and adjust their lives in order to become something that others can live with? Such goals are built on the assumption that sameness is more desirable than difference, that certain kinds of bodies are more valuable than others. In its pursuit of a 'good result', rehabilitation may neglect the person as an embodied subjectivity, it may ignore the possibility of the body as a lived experience. Rehabilitation, in the full sense of the term, may not be possible within the paradigm of scientific medicine.

The narratives of the men and women in this book cover an enormous range of responses and reactions. Although many of the informants in this study may have couched their narratives in terms that are conventional within the rehabilitative vernacular, others used no such accessible terms to identify issues within their own self-project. The new sense of self as part of rehabilitation after injury is built as part of a process of exploring innovative social forms. Just as 'finding oneself' after divorce may involve exploring new forms of step-parenting in modern life (Giddens 1991, p. 33), the reconstitution of self-identity after bodily change may involve negotiation with new forms of disability identity raised in response to the disability movement in recent years. In late modernity, however, a person with severe bodily alterations may explore a huge range of options for reconstitution which may bear no relationship at all to conventional categories of disability identity. Diverse continents may be explored and negotiated in an on-going reflexive project of the self. Although dominant for a time, the medical model of rehabilitation is but one opportunity amongst many. The optimism suggested by this study for new possibilities of bodily expression must also be tempered by a recognition of the reality that these people have experienced. Biomedicine has a powerful influence on all bodies, and people with severe bodily damage are doubly constrained by its power. Rehabilitation, as a specialty within medicine, is heir to the biomedical legacy. People with the type of severe and permanent bodily paralyses addressed in this study have spent many months, even years, in rehabilitative contexts. Even those few informants who have avoided residential rehabilitation do not escape the influence of this particular orientation on the body. The vulnerability of damaged bodies, and the continual necessity to appeal to biomedically oriented agencies for assistance or access to other services, sustain a person's reliance on biomedicine and may serve to suppress other, more optimistic, possibilities.

METHODOLOGY

The first part of this chapter explored a variety of ways that the body has been conceptualised in theory. Although some theoretical approaches are more dogmatic than others, all perspectives arise from different ontological positions which influence the nature of the body as it is seen. Throughout history scholars and researchers have approached the body in terms of their preconceptions; their explorations have often revealed that which was necessary to prove their contentions. The body has been shaped and moulded to reflect different purposes and to fit with particular social needs. Particular views of the body, confirmed by anatomical examination and the experimental method, have enhanced the power of medical science and reproduced the 'truth' of biological conceptions of the body.

The foundationalist and anti-foundationalist positions have dominated sociology. The anti-foundationalist position has arisen in large part as a critique of the positivism of the biomedical conception of the body. The problems created by the dual approach to the body within sociology and the strong reconciliatory movement to overcome the dichotomous positions have been discussed earlier in this chapter. It is to the more specific issue of research perspectives and methodologies that the next section of the chapter is directed. Yet here again it seems we cannot escape the influence of positivist approaches associated with medical knowledge or the polarised positions characteristic of sociological theory.

Research in the social sciences has long been characterised by the

qualitative or quantitative distinction. Quantitative, positivist perspectives involve a foundational epistemology, qualitative approaches
are associated with anti-foundationalism. Quantitative techniques fit
with key features of the medico-scientific approach characterised by
its perceived objectivity, the replicability of findings, the empirical
validation of theory, and implicit in this, its self-correcting nature
(Krathwohl 1985, p. 24). But in imagining that the social world can
be trapped like a butterfly and pinned to a board for investigation,
such researchers may do grave disservice to the rich complexities of
the human social life.

While these features may have served to legitimate social science
research in the eyes of people more versed in the natural sciences,
the real issue between the natural and the social sciences lies in the
relationship of the research to the object being studied. Citing
Giddens (1976), Cohen & Manion (1989, p. 26) note, 'Social science
[. . .] stands in a subject–subject relation to its field of study, not
a subject-object relation; it deals with a pre-interpreted world in
which the meanings given by active subjects actually enter the actual
constitution or production of the world.'

In describing qualitative research methods in relation to quantitative methods, Bryman (1984, pp. 77–8) states,

> The *sine qua non* is a commitment to seeing the social world from the
> point of view of the actor [. . .] There is a simultaneous expression
> of preference for a contextual understanding so that behaviour is to be
> understood in the context of meaning systems employed by a particular
> group or society [. . .] Qualitative research is deemed to be much more
> fluid and flexible than quantitative research in that it emphasises dis-
> covering novel or unanticipated findings and the possibility of altering
> research plans in response to such serendipitous occurrences.

It is these issues that lie at the heart of the quantitative/qualitative
debate within the social sciences. While quantitative methods are
seen to produce objective, value-free knowledge, qualitative methods
are seen to yield no more than subjective, value-laden accounts.
Questions of validity, reliability and objectivity are alleged to differ-
entiate the perspectives. Aligned against each other in these terms,
the two approaches are reduced to competing research modalities
within the social sciences.

However, the notion of what constitutes objective knowledge is
itself problematic, and is made even more critical by issues raised
by postmodern thought (Baum 1993, p. 11). Can human beings ever
achieve any form of knowledge that is independent of their own
subjective construction while they are the agents through which
knowledge is perceived and experienced (Morgan & Smircich 1980,

p. 493)? Objectivity is itself a highly relational concept. Human beings do not merely respond to the world, they actively create and make the world. This on-going, continually changing process defies external observation and measurement: world building must be investigated from within the subject of study using techniques that are appropriate to that task. The researcher should not be exempt from similar scrutiny (Plummer 1995, p. 12).

The sharply drawn, contrasting positions associated with research methodologies resemble the dual positions that have bedevilled social theory, and may be similarly unproductive. Clearly the polarisation of quantitative and qualitative methodologies has been a serious impediment to the development of an adequate methodology in the social sciences, yet the merits and weaknesses of one approach in relation to the other still engage the attention of many scholars (Strauss 1987; Daly & Willis 1990; Minichiello et al. 1990; Patton 1990). Allegiance to either one or the other position has deflected scholars from consideration of more critical issues. Preoccupation with methods highlights the technical aspects of the research while obscuring the infrastructural assumptions upon which the research is based.

Just as recognition of the problems associated with the dual positions in sociological theory has stimulated moves toward integration, the problems associated with the parochialism of the quantitative/qualitative divisions have provoked a similar movement for methodological diversity (Turner et al. 1993). Like all tools, research methodologies must fit the task, not determine the questions and outcomes of social inquiry. The quality of research rests on the appropriateness of its methods rather than its conformity to methodological orthodoxy (Patton 1990, p. 39).

Awareness of the problems inherent in research in general, however, does not guarantee immunity from problems in a specific project. Issues raised by the particular nature of the research for *Remaking the Body* require identification and some discussion.

An exploration of embodiment must utilise a methodology that maximises the informant's point of view, and captures this information in context. While recognising the principle of methodological diversity and being aware of the importance of methodological suitability, the research for this book has proceeded largely within a general framework informed by qualitative methodology (Bryman 1984, pp. 77–8).

Every research project is made up of issues, individuals and experiences that the researcher considers important enough to investigate. Inclusion and, more importantly, exclusion—issues that have been left out or perceived as irrelevant or insignificant—are, in effect, political acts with fundamental implications for the development of knowledge. This is, of course, true of all research, not only of this study.

The advantages of participant observation as a method of engaging with people as collaborators rather than passive informants in a research study were well established in Whyte's early study of urban communities in Chicago (Whyte 1955). In an earlier study (Seymour 1989), I engaged in participant observation over a three-month period in a spinal rehabilitation unit, in addition to extensive data collection outside the institution. Because of this recent experience, I have dispensed with the participant observational component in this new study, although I believe the technique to be essential to this type of research endeavour. The insights gained from this earlier study have been invaluable in helping me understand the experiences of the new informants in this current study. Although this study arises directly out of the previous study, it is significantly different. The focus of this study, though continuing to acknowledge the strong influence of the institution, directs its attention to the broader social context in which attitudes arise and have their impact on the embodiment of men and women.

In her study of torture, Scarry invites us to consider not only the difficulties associated with comprehending 'the atrocities one's own body, muscle and bone structure can inflict on oneself', but also the difficulties one has in comprehending another person's experience of bodily pain (1985, p. 48). A thoughtful researcher may come to imagine how it feels not to feel, but only a person who has experienced sensory loss can know exactly. A sensitive interviewer may suspect that certain aspects of personal relationships may be difficult for a woman who has suffered visible bodily alterations, but the woman alone can tell us what these losses actually mean in terms of her embodied self. No matter how intuitive, no one can ever really know how another person feels. No one can ever know what a particular bodily change means to the integrity of a person's embodiment. No one can fully understand another person's loss. People's feelings, their experiences, the manner in which they perceive that their physical bodily losses have influenced their lives are the data for this study. There is no wiser knowledge, no 'more correct' version of the situation lurking behind the informants' reality.

Yet the body 'lives' in a social context. While the experience of the lived body is personal and in a sense unique, the body is situated in a social context and is subject to its categories. It is through these social categories that the body is revealed in both a phenomenological and a social sense. Thus chapters in this book are devoted to appearance, social routines and relationships, sport and physicality, sexuality, and bodily continence. These domains are key contexts for bodily activities. Exploration of established categories for viewing

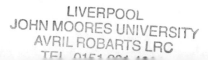

and managing the body presents avenues through which the body is made more accessible. By listening to the paralysed person we may begin to understand the impact of social categories in light of the bodily losses concerned.

In this study randomness—a desirable characteristic in some research design—must be sacrificed in favour of 'snowball sampling' (Minichiello et al. 1990, p. 198). Damaged bodies expose the relationship between the lived body and the influence of society. The only people who can contribute to this understanding are people with extensive bodily loss. A chain of introduction developed from one informant to the next. In many ways, of course, this referral system is not ideal. I believe, however, that the specific needs of the project justify this method.

The principal research theme—the processes involved in remaking the body after severe change or loss—was made clear to my inform- ants at the time of my initial interview request. This overarching theme was couched in terms of characteristic features of conventional masculinity and femininity. Themes such as appearance, sexuality, relationships, bladder and bowel management, motherhood, father- hood, and sport were raised in each interview. Some informants responded with passion to particular themes, others initially down- played the impact of social categories only to acknowledge their significance at a later stage in the discussion. We live in a sexist society, and so many of the interviews reflected the same opacity about the presence and impact of gender in everyday life. It is a function of its very taken-for-grantedness that gender is so difficult to identify. People feel its presence, but cannot identify the obstacles it puts before them.

In an initial conversation, informants discussed with me the most convenient time and place for the interview to take place. With the exception of one interview conducted in my office, I drove to my informants' choice of venue. Although I perceived no particular importance in this practical activity at the time, it is clearly significant to note that although I interviewed eleven women in their homes and only one woman in her workplace, I interviewed eight men in their workplaces, one in a city hotel while drinking beer, one in my office and only two in their homes. The location of the interview has already revealed dramatic differences in the social roles of men and women before a word is spoken. Apart from this strong statement of gender difference, the opportunity, in all but the two instances mentioned, to enter the private worlds of the informants provided extremely useful additional evidence for this study, rein- forcing the verbal points or sometimes providing me with a clue that a particular issue needed more exploration (Kellehear 1993, pp. 115–39). But although all of the men and women in this study chose the location of the interview, the implications associated with setting and location must not be ignored. The vulnerability of women when interviewed within a domestic context has been sensitively discussed by Finch (1984) and Koutroulis (1993, p. 88), and is an important consideration for this study. Far from being neutral environments, the space and setting in which the research takes place are integral to the knowledge that is produced (Minichiello et al. 1990, pp. 200–2).

Many of the informants expressed gratitude for the opportunity to talk about issues that are 'best not talked about' in the usual course of everyday life. Although issues related to bladder and bowel management and sexuality have taken on paramount importance in these people's lives, they are not issues that are commonly raised in everyday conversation. Yet this talk is research data. The express purpose of the discussion about intimate issues was to produce material for research. People with disabled bodies are vulnerable to exploitation by others in many aspects of their lives (Albrecht 1992; Deegan & Brooks 1985; Dovey & Gaffram 1987; Hevey 1992; Lonsdale 1990; Oliver 1990; Smith & Smith 1991). Although this project was essentially no different from any other research project, the susceptibility of the informants in this study is heightened by the particular nature of the material. Although all the informants participated willingly in the study, often initiating the topic and volunteering the information, with some taking advantage of the invitation to edit parts of the material that had been recorded during the interview, I am aware that the specific nature of the inquiry involved in this project makes the informants especially vulnerable.

However it is the very issue of embarrassment associated with discussion of these topics that reinforces the sensitive nature of such bodily activities and compounds the problems that disruption to these aspects of the body may bring. Privacy has conferred on these issues immunity from scrutiny. Yet these activities are critical to our social and personal well-being. The sensitive and private nature of these issues has justified their exclusion from, or at best cursory consideration in, rehabilitation programs for too long. The full reconstitution of the embodied self after bodily disruption can never be complete without specific attention to these critical aspects of bodily activity and self-identity.

The quality of information gained in an interview involving sensitive issues depends more than ever on the researcher's ability to establish rapport and a trusting relationship with the informant. Successful research outcomes thus derive directly from these personal attributes and from the quality of the interaction that develops between the informant and the researcher. Not surprisingly, these two characteristics provoke great academic scepticism. When compared with the more overtly disciplined and rigorous techniques of quantitative methodologies, qualitative interviews may appear subjective, idiosyncratic, and of little value in generating reliable and valid research data. Can the god of objectivity be served by a method that depends on such nebulous qualities as rapport, trust and respect to support an interaction context of data collection?

It is certainly not my intention to strengthen the polarities by perpetuating the on-going debate about the advantages and disadvantages of qualitative compared with quantitative methodologies. Suffice to say that this debate has been discussed lucidly and well by many scholars (Daly & Willis 1990; Minichiello et al. 1990; Patton 1990; Strauss 1987). For my part, I am alert to the potential for distortion that can occur in such a personalised context, but I am no less concerned about the bias that may inform the design of less discursive, more detached methodologies. Similarly, I am aware that the dangers of exploitation may be heightened, not eradicated, by an attempt to create a more equal relationship between the researcher and the researched (Williams 1988, p. 110).

Beyond the more instrumental concerns associated with the process of the research project just discussed, what role does the researcher play in the construction of the data?

It is important, at this point, for the researcher to acknowledge her own disability. Although not of the same dramatic or catastrophic nature as the disabilities experienced by the men and women in this study, a long-standing progressive condition has nevertheless extorted considerable bodily losses with, no doubt, concomitant changes in self-identity in order to reconcile painful and visibly deformed body parts with social conventions of femininity, age, class and career aspirations. It was made clear to me by many of the informants that, in their eyes, the disability legitimated my right to conduct the research. This, added to my work experience in rehabilitative situations and previous research in the area, seemed to confirm that I had paid my dues in terms of commitment to the area. In everyday life we respond to people on the basis of their external body. In this particular context, my own visible body seems to have played a more direct role in the generation of research material.

Raising this issue goes beyond mere indulgent self-revelation. Traditional forms of writing sociology hide the role of the writer; what is written is displayed as if it were disconnected from the processes that made it possible (Wynne 1988, p. 103). Putting oneself into the picture—exposing issues related to the researcher that may influence the nature of the data—is clearly critical to the research project. If the 'objectivity' of research can be compromised by selection of research location (Finch 1984; Koutroulis 1993, p. 88) and time (Minichiello et al. 1990, p. 200), then failure to consider the role of the researcher in the creation of a research project represents a serious dereliction of accountability. Other more general characteristics are embedded in all research, yet are seldom acknowledged.

Gender, age, social class, prestige, ethnic identity, expertise, friendship are salient variables in all interactional contexts; in the context of the researcher–informant relationship these issues become very powerful. Critical self-reflection on the part of the researcher is an essential component of the research project.

The production of social science knowledge about the world is itself a social activity (Woolgar & Ashmore 1988, p. 1). We reflexively create reality from what we take to be the documents of that reality; the talk of others is one such document (Wynne 1988, p. 103). Discursive processes are involved in the construction of what comes to be seen as coherent knowledge (Game 1991, p. 7). These points have been raised earlier in this chapter. The act of writing up research materials is a critical activity. Unstructured interviews were used in this study in order to explore what disrupted embodiment meant to the men and women and to allow them to tell their stories in their own way. But how much is the researcher implicated in the knowledge process, in the writing of culture (Game 1991, p. 7)? In order to create an accessible account of the extensive research data, the researcher must select extracts from this material. What guides this selection? Parts are taken from their original context and inserted into a new document in terms of the researcher/writer's interpretation. No matter how conscientiously this process is conducted, it must distort the original meaning of the documents, assuming of course that they have an original meaning that is fixable (Wynne 1988, p. 106).

It seems that putting oneself in the picture—reflecting on the role of the researcher as well as the researched—presents a Pandora's box of 'methodological horrors' (Wynne 1988, p. 114). No matter how genuine the commitment of the researcher to the integrity of the informant's reality, the outcome must always be the same: in effect special status is assumed for one's own analysis. One may claim that the research is dedicated to documenting the features that the men and women use to produce their own stories; but the act of analysis is predicated on 'seeing behind' the informants' own accounts, on demonstrating features that are not visible to the people themselves (Wynne 1988, p. 113), on producing a privileged representation of social reality (Game 1991, p. 7), a better understanding of the informants' reality than they have themselves.

This raises serious methodological issues about all research. The empiricist view that facts 'speak for themselves' is clearly a nonsense (Blumer 1982, p. 92). Although the 'work' involved in the production of conventional empiricist accounts is usually concealed, no project can be free of the a priori assumptions of the researcher. Research data

are those that are recorded (Wynne 1988, p. 17), they are a visible
record of people's stories. The final written product of the research
endeavour is a far more complex synthesis of diverse factors oriented
to this material, but invisible to the process. To imagine otherwise is
to engage with the delusion embedded in the debates on objectivity.
Although this issue is critical, the research enterprise need not be
diminished by it. As discussed earlier, the issue of objectivity has been
a vexed question in social science research, a durable legacy of the
positivist past. Yet questions of objectivity are only important if one
believes that they are important, and that such a position is possible
to achieve (Wynne 1988, p. 121). In acknowledging the unrecorded,
invisible influences that constitute the research project, a researcher is
merely making overt those factors that are covert in all research
endeavours. All research must take into account the factors involved
in its own production (Latour 1988, p. 166; Plummer 1995, p. 13).

My own roles as a person with a visible disability, as a former
health professional, as a social scientist and as a woman are just
some of the more obvious factors that have influenced the selection
of informants, the process of the interview, the analysis of the
material and the theoretical underpinnings of the project. No story,
however, remains true for ever (Plummer 1995, p. 170). Time,
changed circumstances, rehabilitative progress and ageing are just
some of the factors that have influenced the informants since they
first told me their stories. The men and women may not recognise
every aspect of their own story at this or any future point of time.
However, we cannot assume that the reader of this study will be a
passive recipient of the text. Readers, too, are active interpreters of
what they read, and will reconstitute the substance of the work to
suit their socio-cultural circumstances (Colquhoun 1993, p. 71) as
well as a range of other factors. Thus informants, readers and the
researcher bring diverse perspectives and interpretations to the research project. What appears in this study is an illuminating,
engaging account of disruption and re-embodiment. It is an account
of the work of twenty-four people in restoring their bodies after
severe injury, an interweaving of the phenomenological body and
social discourse in the reconstitution of the self. The task will
continue for these women and men long after this book has been
published: this research represents the insights of these people in the
process of remaking their fragmented, embodied selves in a context
of great uncertainty and risk. In directly confronting the comfortable
certainties provided by the theoretical and methodological positions
of the past, this study will encourage health workers, rehabilitation
professionals and social scientists to explore the more hazardous,
but also more expansive, possibilities presented by and to the body
in the new world.

2 Appearance and body image

R ecent years have seen the development of an aesthetics of the body in consumer culture. While the body has always been susceptible to aesthetic concerns, in the past in Western societies it remained a project for elite court groups or for a high bourgeois culture. In contemporary society the body as a personal project has become the pursuit of a mass audience (Turner 1994, p. xiii). A vast array of dietary, slimming, exercise and cosmetic products point to the significance of appearance and bodily presentation within late capitalist society (Featherstone 1987, p. 18).

THE BODY PROJECT: STRUCTURAL FORCES AND HUMAN EMBODIMENT

Consumer culture provides a multitude of stylised images of the body. The surface of the body has become the target for advertising goods, technologies and services in a consumer society, but in the process the appearance of the body has become more susceptible to stigmatisation. If the appearance of the body can be shaped and changed by the unlimited consumption of goods, men and women must bear responsibility for being other than what they could be. Since body image plays a key role in the evaluation of the self in society, men and women work on their bodies in order to enhance their body image for themselves and for others.

The notion of a body project, however, goes far beyond the relatively simple creation of a socially valued, objective bodily presentation. Notions of the stable, objective bodies of men and of women, derived from biomedicine, were based on male-dominated ways of thought. Ideas of normality and abnormality rested on the sharply drawn male–female dichotomy. Sociological understanding centres on the idea that while we are born either male or female, masculinity and femininity are social products. The patriarchal gender order creates particular understandings, practices and definitions concerning men and women. Connell uses the term 'hegemonic masculinity' (1987, p. 183) to describe the stylised and impoverished form of masculinity that dominates gender relations. Connell borrows Gramsci's use of the term 'hegemony' by which he refers to social ascendancy achieved by the impact of cultural processes on private lives. Hegemonic ascendancy is achieved not by violent means, but by the power embedded in cultural practices. Religious doctrine and practices, the media, cultural texts, image structures and policies are powerful coercive forces. Hegemonic masculinity is constructed in relation to various other subordinated masculinities, as well as in relation to women.

Femininity, although by no means as authoritative as hegemonic masculinity, is nevertheless clearly defined. Connell uses the term 'emphasised femininity' to identify the form of femininity that is 'defined around compliance with subordination and is oriented to accommodating the interests and desires of men' (1987, p. 183). Hegemonic masculinity is heterosexual, and is characterised by power, authority, aggression and technical competence (Connell 1987, pp. 186–7). Complementing hegemonic masculinity are the characteristics embodied in emphasised femininity—sociability, sexual passivity, acceptance of domesticity and motherhood (Connell 1987, p. 187). Hegemonic masculinity must continually act to subvert other masculinities, notably the key form of subordinated masculinity, homosexuality. In contrast, all forms of femininity are constructed in relation to the overall subordination of women to men. This fact, Connell claims, limits the scope of women to assert power over other women.

These constructions of masculinity and femininity are promoted as cultural ideals. Emphasised femininity is the substance of the mass media, advertisements and daytime television. Such extensive propagation obscures other forms of femininity as experienced by 'spinsters, lesbians, unionists, prostitutes, mad women, rebels and maiden aunts, manual workers, midwives and witches' (Connell 1987, p. 188) and, importantly, women with disabilities. The patriarchal gender order requires differentness, but within the bounds of complementarity and rigid rules, and thus categories of gender are limited. Is it possible to be creative in the face of dominant gender ideologies that promote certain forms of masculinity and femininity?

Can men and women transcend what is expected of their gender? The experiences of the men and women in this study undermine and subvert ideas of what is normal for a man, or what a normal woman should look like. This study focuses on the shift from the confining, single, objective body of biomedical and patriarchal discourse—the masculine body or the feminine body—to the expansive possibilities of embodied subjectivities.

The on-going body project involves corporeality or bodiliness as the experientiality of the body (Turner 1994, p. xii). Appearance and body image are fundamentally related to embodiment, to the fact that human beings are embodied social agents. Human beings not only have a body, but also actively engage in the development of their bodies over their lifetimes; human beings are bodies (Turner 1994, p. xi). Modern selfhood is intimately connected with the body (Synnott 1993; Shilling 1993). In exploring how the embodied social actors in this study actively engage in the project of remaking their visibly damaged bodies, this chapter will illuminate aspects of the dynamics of body image in social contexts.

Although the men and women in this study have experienced severe alteration to aspects of their bodies, other significant aspects of their bodies remain. Despite the losses, these people are still able to use their bodies in order to see, to listen, to feel, to smell and to act about and on their bodies. The disruption that the men and women have experienced has emphasised the taken-for-grantedness of many aspects of everyday life which they now find challenging, but they still have a body which they experience. The crisis may have changed the way they are able to respond to events, but their bodies still feel, and over time they will devise new ways to respond to their experiences. Although different, the experience of the body is still authentic. The men and women actively engage in reshaping their bodies. It is through their embodied experiences that true rehabilitation takes place.

Appearance is a conspicuous aspect of the self. The external body presents itself boldly to the world. It is impossible to hide the external body from the view and appraisal of others. Women in some Muslim countries may veil their bodies from the scrutiny of all but their family, yet this strategy is itself a source of evidence for further assumptions. The outside of the body is a public property. Others see the external body and may make assumptions about it with or without our approval or knowledge. Not only can people make assumptions about the bodies of others from these passing appraisals, but also many people feel confident that appearance provides sufficient evidence of interior personal qualities, that external appearance relates directly to the essential nature of the person. Dominant gender ideologies promote particular forms of masculine and feminine appearance. The social construction of masculinity and femininity exaggerates the differences and emphasises the essential complementarity between men and women upon which patriarchy depends (Connell & Dowsett 1992, p. 73). Although appearance is a critical element of self-identity for both men and women, there is no doubt that women fare much less well in terms of body evaluation than men. The appearance of the external body is critical in the dominant construction of femininity (Coward 1984; Game & Pringle 1979; Gilbert & Taylor 1991; Pringle 1983). Being attractive to men is implicit in emphasised femininity. Women's self-identity and their life opportunities may be decided by their appearance, the evaluation of which is usually done by men.

Awareness of this continual process of scrutiny and evaluation encourages men and women to employ an enormous range of strategies to attract or deflect other people's attention to or from aspects of their bodies. However, no matter what consumer goods are chosen or which strategies are used to alter the body, an external body image remains—the appearance may be different, unusual or challenging, but it is a body nonetheless, and it can still be seen by others. Because others will act on the basis of their appraisal of a person based on his or her external appearance, other people are important agents in the development and maintenance, and in the destruction, of self-esteem. Since appearance is the evidence upon which their appraisal is based, external appearance is a critical element of self-identity.

Notions of beauty, attractiveness, fashion and slimness, characteristics of the external body, dominate conventional constructions of femininity. The externality of this construction exacerbates women's vulnerability to others. Body shape, size, contours and postures emit strong social messages, which are reinforced by clothing. Style, texture, cut and colour of clothing reveal clues about how people see themselves and their place in the world. Choice is heavily influenced by the inevitability of evaluation by others. Far from being a creative aspect of the self, fashion can be seen as an instrument of alienation from the self (Emberley 1988, p. 49). While claiming to express individuality, fashion invites people to conform to the market uniformity of seasonal products. The manner in which we drape and decorate our body is not an expression of individuality but rather an acceptance and collusion with prevailing ideas, an 'anchoring of our bodies, particularly the bodies of women, into specific positions, and parts of the body in the line of gaze' (Sawchuk 1988, pp. 62–3). Yet anti-fashion discourse may be motivated by an intention to repress women's potential for subversive bodily expression and return women to the proper sphere of the home (Sawchuk 1988, p. 67). While it is clear that the appearance of the body reflects structural forces, bodily aesthetics are critical to embodiment. These forces are formidable, but women are not mere victims of structural ideologies operating through the fashion and cosmetics industries. Although women may employ the products of consumerism, the body project is part of human embodiment. Human beings use their bodies to create their appearance as part of their embodied selves. While body images may conform to conventional categories of appearance, the potential for creative and subversive resistance to prevailing conventions is always present.

'To be an adult male is distinctly to occupy space, to have a physical presence in the world' (Connell 1983, p. 33). A man's presence is dependent upon the promise of power which he embodies (Berger 1972, p. 45). Sport is a critical vehicle of conventional masculine body appearance (Sabo & Runfola 1980). The embedding of power within the male body is reinforced by the appropriation of sport by consumer culture (Hargreaves 1986, p. 10). It is the body that constitutes the most striking symbol as well as the material core of sporting activity (Hargreaves 1986, p. 12). However, the body not only symbolises power relations, power is literally incorporated into the body (Hargreaves 1986, p. 13). Participation in sport changes the body; masculine ideas become embedded into the body—embodiment, quite literally, occurs (Connell, 1983, p. 33). To be masculine means to embody force and competence. Force and competence are the physical manifestations of social relations that define men as holders of power and women as subordinate. Through the constant exercising undertaken by boys, and the social constraints that inhibit girls from similar activities, these statements become embedded into the body, not just in mental body images, but in the very feel and texture of the body, its attitudes, its muscular tensions, its surfaces (Connell 1983, p. 38).

Over time the bodies of men and women are physically transformed by the social structures of gender. Discussions of male physicality give little or no account of the impact of social ideas on individual practices (Hargreaves 1986, p. 2). Male bones and muscles are strong because men have been encouraged to use their bodies. Through history, men have been encouraged to see themselves in particular ways. Men's minds have internalised particular social messages and expectations about the male body. Such messages stimulate the spinal nerves to activate the voluntary muscles that move the joints and bones of the skeleton in specific ways. Men have been encouraged to extend their bodies to the limit in combat, agriculture, construction, defence and tournaments and contests of all kinds. Muscle action enhances the flow of blood which supplies oxygen and nutrients to the bones, which stimulates bone growth and strength. The critical relationship between ideas and actions makes it difficult to separate social ideas from their embodiment. Ideas about masculinity encourage the kinds of activities that build the musculoskeletal system; the strength and the size of men's musculoskeletal systems encourage assumptions about the kinds of activities men should do. This circularity guarantees the reproduction both of ideas and practices and, more critically, ensures the continuation of the patriarchal gender order and its enshrined inequalities. Many men fall short of the physical dimensions of hegemonic masculinity, yet such is the power of the patriarchal gender order that all men will benefit.

DISABILITY AND BODILY EXPRESSION

The preceding discussion of appearance in relation to categories of emphasised femininity and hegemonic masculinity may appear to draw a picture of women as passive victims of fashion and consumerism and men as dupes of the ideology of sport. This discussion was necessary to acknowledge these powerful stereotypes, not to collude with the status quo. The men and women in this study have learned particular interpretations of their bodily experiences and specific ways of thinking about their bodies since birth. They have embodied social ideas and these ideas have become the substance of their consciousness, the tools by which they evaluate themselves and others. But although social categories are laid down in bodies, they may be destabilised. The crises experienced by the men and women in this study disrupted years of careful socialisation. The anarchy of the paralysed and disordered body challenges social categories and forces the person to engage his or her body in the active, on-going process of re-embodiment.

Many of the informants seem to be reproducing, rather than challenging or transcending, conventional forms of masculine or feminine bodily expression. While it may seem that many of the men and women attempt to recreate their former selves, or remake their bodies in terms of dominant ideas about male or female bodies, it is important to remember that their bodies, like all bodies, are in a process of change. The informants are all at different stages of their re-embodiment, and this research captures only a part of this continuing process. The vulnerability of these damaged bodies to institutional narratives, the necessity for dependence on others, and the lure of the past act to discourage innovation. While conventional constructions of masculine and feminine bodies may guide the process of re-embodiment for many of the informants, over time the experience of visibly damaged bodies in everyday social interaction may point to different kinds of bodies which are less tied to the male–female dichotomy and its associated concepts of normality and abnormality. While there is little evidence of a fully developed postmodern body amongst the informants in this study, many of the men and women demonstrate that they have moved well beyond the confinements of the unified body of formal rehabilitative discourse in their own embodied rehabilitation—in their re-embodiment.

Body maintenance tasks—hair care, facial management, grooming and clothing the body—take up an inordinate part of our lives, yet these activities are so commonplace that we seldom stop to account for the time, energy and anxiety we devote to them. Bodily appearance, maintenance and image construction require constant analysis, evaluation and technical skill if we are to display an external appearance that is congruent with the way we see ourselves and the way we wish others to see us. The continuous body work in which we engage throughout our everyday lives is hidden from view unless some event or issue compels us to acknowledge it.

The Western commercial world offers such an abundance of clothing that we seldom stop to think that most clothing is designed and constructed with certain assumptions about the human body in mind. That the body will be upright is taken for granted; that wearers will be able to fasten any number of buttons, hooks, laces and zippers with their hands is assumed to be unproblematic. The body, especially a woman's body, will have a slender waist, certain dimensions and relationships between upper and lower body, and particular shapes of legs, arms, neck and chest. Although clothing may make fewer demands of men's bodies, nevertheless men's formal wear requires particular shapes and bodily postures for its full effect.

Choice of clothing for a man or woman with a disability may be severely limited. Not only will the practical aspects of getting dressed be difficult, but once these obstacles have been eliminated, the men and women are left to select from a very narrow range of choices to satisfy their changed body and disordered sense of self. The impact of bodily loss may be compounded by the need to cover the damaged body with clothing that is at odds with the embodied self. Clothing may seriously exacerbate the experience of disembodiment for people with serious paralysis.

The men and women often stressed the importance of looking like other people, especially in the competitive world of work. Yet the need to wear garments that can be managed by hands with limited movement, or clothes that can accommodate splints, calipers, drainage bottles and the other impedimenta of disability may make this goal hard to attain. Certainly those men and women who live with an able-bodied partner or parent have a better chance of being able to select clothing from a wider range of styles, and dressing may be facilitated by a care attendant for those people who live on their own. But the bodily changes impose a particular style of dressing on most of the people in this study, which is often profoundly felt.

Loss of sensation means that the mere act of sitting in a wheelchair or lying in a bed becomes a hazardous activity. The paralysed person is not able to move his or her body as other people do, even at rest, and because he or she cannot feel that damage is occurring, a pressure sore can develop very quickly. For this reason, soft pants of the tracksuit variety are most often chosen to avoid the possibility of inadvertently sitting on creased trousers, thick seams, studs or any of the other design details of fashion clothing. Similarly, feet that have lost movement and sensation are susceptible to knocking and burning as well as to circulatory disturbances such as chilblains. Choice of footwear is curtailed by the need to protect the feet from these dangers. Apart from these restrictions, many of the men and women in this study are unable to bend down to put shoes on their feet, much less to tie the laces.

Weakness or paralysis of the abdominal muscles is also a common issue for the people in this study. This muscle loss creates a characteristic pot-bellied appearance which many of the men and women find particularly distressing. The body appears shortened because the normally strong abdominal muscles no longer support the chest and rib cage. Since so much dressing for both men and women depends on the presence of a waist, this loss creates problems for people wishing to look like everyone else, and to be able to select their clothing from the same sources. A loose shirt or blouse hanging over the top of soft pants is the most common way both men and women overcome this weakness.

Wasting of the leg muscles often results in a stick-legged appearance. This, again, means that many people choose to wear long, loose pants, rather than jeans, tailored trousers, shorts or skirts. Development of the muscles that are supplied by the intact nerves above the level of the lesion is actively encouraged for all people with paraplegia or similar conditions. The aim of such activities is to strengthen the muscles of the upper back, shoulders and neck in order that these parts of the body can carry out additional functions of lifting and transferring the lower parts of the body which are no longer capable of movement. Energetic and carefully planned activities involving muscle-building work of the upper trunk, shoulder and arm muscles are an important functional task of rehabilitation, but these activities also create a powerful physical definition of masculinity which has the potential to override other losses the paralysed man may have incurred in relation to conventional presentations of masculinity (Seymour 1989, p. 114). Clothing, particularly men's sporting clothing, sits well on this developed upper torso, and such dressing serves to deflect attention from those other parts of the man's body that do not work so well. Conventional femininity does not offer women with disabilities a similarly convenient category to reconstruct their bodily appearance. While the functional advantages of a well-developed upper body are clearly the same for men and for women, strong shoulders and arms do not fit with dominant constructions of femininity. Women who succeed in building their upper body in this way may risk losing more than they gain in terms of 'unfeminine' bodily shape and definitions (Lupton 1994, pp. 39–40). Despite the recent achievements of Bev Francis and other women athletes, body building is still not considered a feminine activity. Conventional femininity cannot incorporate such overt displays of bodily strength.

Most of the men and women in this study (introduced to readers on pp. 14–15) have experienced a profound change in their appearance. Those men and women who have had their disability since birth may not have experienced the sudden, dramatic alteration in their bodily appearance that most of the informants have had to manage, but their bodies have progressively developed in a manner that fails to conform to conventional presentations of masculine and feminine appearance. How have the men and women in this study experienced these dramatic changes in their appearance? These people live in a body that confronts masculine and feminine stereotypes about appearance. How have they pursued their lives in a society that places such high value on physical appearance?

Appearance and crisis

'Looks' were always extremely important to Frances: 'I had never worried about exposing my body. I had walked around in bathers or just nothing all my life because my body had always done exactly what I wanted it to. I never had to diet, it was always just fine. I knew I had what was termed a good body.' Ian learned early in his training in the armed forces that: 'If you want to be an officer you've got to look like one. I knew that if I wanted to compete with the rest of the world I needed to look like other people.' Appearance and the presentation of her body has always been important to Joy. Her first work as an adolescent was as a photographic model. Her desire to display her body in a way that satisfies her ideas about herself is no less strong since her accident, although these appearances are much more difficult to execute. Frances, too, had been a model. She says:

> I would regard myself as what would be classed as a 'natural person'. Although I had been a model in my late teens, and I

*had worn make-up, and knew how to apply it, I had rejected it
a couple of years later and not worn it since. Appearance for me
was based on a whole body image rather than just portrayal of
the face as such. I suppose I had been lucky in that I was very
confident about my body because I had been tall and slim and
good at sports. I had this feeling that my body could do anything
I wanted it to.*

Ron has 'always been a fairly fastidious person and been aware
of the way I dress. I have never liked being dressed like a slob.' Bob
saw himself as 'sporty' before his accident: 'I didn't think that I was
any Elvis Presley, and I was pretty shy, but once I was encouraged
a little bit I went for it. I wasn't a very big person, although I was
quite muscular—I guess from doing a lot of sport. I guess I was
happy with my own body image. I had rippled muscles and stuff
like that.' Although Ruth has had to manage her disabling condition
all her life she says: 'I think that as a kid I was regarded as relatively
attractive. I was slim and trim and, you know, I had a traditionally
attractive body shape. I could wear a bikini, and I thought I looked
pretty flash. I was never short on boyfriends.'

The initial shock to the body caused by the injury or the infection
produces dramatic visible changes to the appearance of the body.
Frances says:

*When I was in intensive care, particularly, I didn't want to look
at myself because I had this image of myself as looking very grey.
I knew that I had lost about two stone in weight. My hair fell
out for a while too—it didn't fall right out, but it thinned. And
so I had this image of myself as this balding, grey person. When
I finally did look at myself in the mirror, I was surprised because
I didn't look as bad as I had expected.*

Bob says: 'I remember that a male nurse used to come in every
morning and measure my thighs and measure my calves, and I
remember him saying one day, "Well, now you have got the skinniest
legs in the ward".'

The issue that remains vivid in Jenny's memory from the early
days of her rehabilitation was related to her hair:

*Hair washing was not seen as something that was required of
the staff. I didn't have a mother there to do it, or anyone like
that, and my partner wasn't—well I didn't have that sort of
relationship. So I managed to get my hair washed about two or
three times in the five weeks that I was there. I had shoulder-
length hair. I was used to washing it every second day. The times*

that I managed to get it washed meant that a staff member had to stay back after hours to do it. It was male nurses who did it—they were more caring and attentive about it actually.

Pam's experience with her hair, although some years before Jenny's experience, was much more positive. Pam says: 'They used to be good about having my hair done. They used to send me into a hairdresser in town with a nurse. It was at their suggestion, not mine. Whether they recognised the importance of this because I was a woman, or whether they recognised it because of me, I don't know.' Clearly Jenny's recollection relates to the initial stage of acute care and Pam's memory is associated with the less difficult second stage of rehabilitation, yet the issue is vivid for each woman. Frances, unlike Jenny, had good experiences in relation to her personal care in the early stages of her illness. She says:

They were very good in intensive care in that they made huge efforts to wash my hair and do things like that, which were almost impossible tasks for someone in a respirator. I had very long hair at the time, but they went to great lengths to help me with physical appearance. They wanted me to wear make-up, but I never wore make-up anyway. I said that it wasn't me to wear make-up, but they were obviously trying to brighten up my appearance.

Unlike Jenny, Pam and Frances, Tina's bodily changes were not sudden. Tina lived in an institution for a large part of her life. She says: 'I had nurses that would do my hair nicely. They really took pride in getting people looking okay. I would ask them to do something for me and they would do that hairstyle, and I would say, "Yes I like that". They were pretty good.' The importance of being able to manage those few aspects of appearance that can be controlled when so many other exterior elements of the body are out of control is, clearly, enormous.

Pam talks about the clothing she wore while she was in the rehabilitation unit:

The common practice was to be in pyjama pants while you were going through all your training because that was simple, and they were washable. I can remember being in these pyjama pants one day when the doctor came in and said, 'Why is she in pyjama pants? That is not good for her'. He thought that I should be fully dressed, but, you see, it was the nurses' easy way out. It was more of an effort, but I was never in pyjama pants after that. I always wore slacks, and I still do.

Frances, too, remembers wearing very big, baggy pants and wearing men's shoes at one stage in order to accommodate the splints and other impedimenta of early rehabilitation. She goes on:

> Then I started to dress myself, but I needed things that I could put on easily. So I went through a phase of tracksuits, which were pretty awful. I asked one of my friends if she could do some shopping for me. She came back with some gloriously bright tracksuits and things, and she said something to me like, 'We realise that it is still important how you look'. I hadn't really thought about it, but she said it so nicely. I had been thinking that it is just important that I get my body moving, and I hadn't thought about that. Once she said that I started thinking, yeah, and facing up to it.

Rebuilding the embodied self after crisis

How does the concept of the body survive such severe disruption in appearance? How do people remake their embodied selves after such crisis and disorder? Society has a readily available model of disabled identity which many people with permanent disabilities may choose to accept. The parameters of this model are strictly defined in terms of the able-bodied world and its domination by particular expressions of masculine and feminine behaviour and appearance. Although this model is readily recognisable, and although it undoubtedly brings comfort to many people, it is a facsimile of real life. The person with the disability is restricted to behaviours and expressions that the able-bodied world can accept. The person may feel unwilling to protest or to rebel for fear of losing the few privileges that the model offers.

Rebuilding the embodied self after such disruption is an extremely difficult task. A person's self-image has been developed over a lifetime in relation to particular social ideas and in terms of a body with certain skills, abilities and appearances. To confront, and to gradually let go of, those aspects of self-identity that now can never be consummated is the most difficult task of rehabilitation. To hang on to the past, though understandable as a protective strategy in the early stages of the crisis, is ultimately counterproductive because it prevents the person from exploring new subjectivities that relate to his or her new body, and to the world within which the person will now live.

Although Bob saw himself as 'sporty' before his accident, he claims that now 'people tend to call me a hippie—I am not sure what I am'. Tina says: 'To tell you the truth, I'm a bit mixed up. I have been trying to analyse why I am like this. I have all these images of myself. Some people see me as a hippie, some people see me as a down-to-earth practical type. People see me in all different ways.' Frances, too, says: 'I have gone through all sorts of phases—of being terribly hippyish—I did that for quite a few years.' It is not surprising to hear these men and women describe themselves in this way. The 'hippie era' of the late sixties and early seventies was a protest against conventional behaviours, forms and appearances. By 'dropping out', men and women expressed their contempt for the prejudices, inconsistencies and hypocrisies of the dominant culture. Experimenting with different social arrangements, sexual behaviours and clothing styles was a significant characteristic of this important time of social questioning. That many 'fellow travellers' rode on the coat-tails of the serious protesters diminishes neither the significance of this time of social unrest nor the genuine desire of the people involved to create a society free of the constraints and conventions of the contemporary society; in fact many of the concerns of the time are reminiscent of those of the postmodern era.

The men and women in this study were not motivated by overt political goals such as these, at least not initially. Their actions are not the product of ethical or moral decisions arising from a social consciousness. The need to confront conventional behaviours was forced upon these men and women by their experience of bodily disruption. The self and the body are inextricable; a disruption to the body inevitably disrupts the embodied self. Yet given this situation, many people have used the crisis to actively engage with and explore their embodiment and in so doing have questioned and challenged conventional categories related to masculinity and femininity in our society. Embodied rehabilitation reconstitutes embodiment.

For some people the crisis presented an opportunity to analyse the taken-for-granted aspects of their previous appearance in order to develop strategies for reconstitution. The facilitative power of conventional categories of masculine appearance may seem to offer an expedient rehabilitative route for some of the men. Ian recognised this early on in his disability and claims that he has used this to improve his rehabilitative chances:

I knew that if I wanted to compete with the rest of the world I needed to look like other people. So I have done a certain amount of repression of my own personality regarding clothes and I play a role where I merge in. It doesn't always work out like that, because underneath it all I am a bit of a rebel, and so sometimes it is only half-way there. But I certainly have been aware of having adequate clothing which looks good, and of coming up with some sort of image close to what other people are doing.

Before her illness, Frances had always been very confident about her body:

I had been tall and slim and good at sports, so I had this feeling that my body could do anything that I wanted it to. So for my body to be like this was obviously cataclysmic. I wasn't worried about what my face would look like, I was worried about how my body would look and my whole appearance. When I finally stood up in front of a full-length mirror, I was pretty horrified. I was obviously very bony, but also the flesh on my legs was just hanging, in particular on my upper thighs—there was sort of nothing there, just bone in the lower part. So that was pretty scary stuff, but at least I consoled myself that I could concentrate more on my facial appearance because I was still in a wheelchair at this stage. But I have always felt a bit awkward because I have to wear lace-up shoes. I can't wear light shoes. I have always had this quandary of how to balance up what I wear. I have tried wearing normal-length skirts below my knee at times with my splints showing, but I feel very uncomfortable, I can't handle it, I have tried, and it just doesn't work for me. Now, ten years on, I wear pants all the time. To put a skirt on I feel absolutely naked. I am glad that I wasn't driven by fashion before my illness, and that I always had what I regarded as my individual style, so it has been much easier for me to be less conforming post-disability and illness than it may have been for other people who were very tied in to fashion cycles. I always used to make my own clothes, and so I chose what I wore and how I wanted to be. There are occasions and workplaces that I am in where I feel if only I could wear a skirt and prove that I am a woman—so that does pass through my mind. In the past I was a person who didn't really care about how I looked because I really didn't have to bother, whereas now I have to think more carefully.

Conformity to existing social categories of appearance may be the most beguiling pathway for people to take, not only because these expressions are known, but also because the approval of others is likely to reward these actions. Exploration of novel expressions of embodiment are likely to be much more difficult since few prior models exist, and society is unlikely to reward the attempts. Alternative expressions are likely to be ignored or devalued. A strategy to diminish the impact of the challenging behaviour of adolescents, for example, is to defer to the temporary nature of such rebellion. Patronising remarks along the lines of 'How nice that so-and-so is brave enough to do this or that' is the way the efforts of many people with intellectual and physical disabilities are dismissed.

Jenny talks of her difficulties in constructing her body image—her sense of wholeness—after her accident:

One thing that was very important was what I wore, how I appeared. At the time I returned home, those sort of tiered, flouncy skirts were in—in the early eighties. I went home and I chucked them all out—all that flouncy, 'in' stuff. I couldn't work out what clothes to wear. It was like being an adolescent, and trying to discover what you look good in. And the troubles of trying things on made it all seem worse. I was lucky in that I was surrounded by all these friends who were aware and sensitive to the issues. I remember going into town with a friend who was a psychologist, and we went through a whole range of stuff about what looked good and what didn't, and what to buy. I had to discover my own presentation. I can remember another friend getting into my wheelchair one day and saying, 'This is what you look like. You don't look like a wheelchair. It's all right, you look nice in a wheelchair'.

Pam, too, had to abandon her previous collection of clothing on her return home after her rehabilitation period. She says:

I suppose in the early days I didn't feel too satisfied about my dressing at all. The most important thing on my mind in those first years was learning to cope with my family. But nevertheless there was a strong sense of concern over the fact that I couldn't wear the sorts of clothes that I liked. I had just made a whole new wardrobe of gorgeous new clothes before the accident, and none of them was any good. I just had to pack up all my wardrobe and give it all away.

Eliminating skirts from their wardrobes seems to be a common strategy for many of the women. Frances has already talked about her avoidance of them. Mary says:

I don't wear skirts because my life has to be geared to getting in and out of a car. When you get into a car your skirt rides up, and when you get out of a car your skirt rides up the other way, and you get out and you are all twisted up. So it's easier to wear trousers. But I like to wear pretty tops. I like my hair to look good. I like to have my trousers with the knife edges coming right down there, not one leg higher than the other, but equal. I like to make sure that my socks go with what I've got on. I have gone through a lot of experimenting with clothes.

Unlike the other women, though, Joy finds wearing long skirts is easier for her. She says:

I really do miss walking around in beautiful clothes. It is important to me to always look good now because if I am pushing along in a chair, with a woman walking along beside me, they are going to look at her first before they look at me. Someone who is walking can offer a lot more to the eye than I can.

Joy regrets that she can no longer wear some of the clothes she would have worn in the past:

I wear skirts most of the time now, whereas before I used to wear jeans occasionally, and look nice. I had a great body, I had a beautiful body. I never had any problems in attracting men at all. I could just about have any man I wanted. Now it's a bit restricted to the clothes that you wear, but I still look good all the time. I like people to say, 'You always look good, Joy, you always dress well'.

Before her accident Joy used to work as a photographic model, often doing naked body shots. She has begun to do some similar work again. She says: 'I am doing modelling now. My friend Harry has taken some photos which they showed on a television channel when I was there the week before last. It is just me, lying on the bed, you can see my bum and my arms. You can't see all of my naked body, but you can see part of it.' While Joy seems comfortable with her new body, Ruth is often shocked when she is confronted with an image of herself as others see her. Clearly her outward appearance does not coincide with the picture she has of herself in her head: 'When I saw a photograph of myself on the television news I was shocked. I said to my son, "Do I walk like that?". He said, innocently, "Yeah, Mum, that's how you walk!". It shocks me still whenever I see it. It just isn't how I imagine I walk.'

People attribute their re-embodiment to different events and issues. Some of the men and women highlight what they see as the worst parts of their bodies, while others seem to disown their bodies. For others, it is the affirmation that comes from others that is the most significant transformational agency. Pam claims that she sees herself now as one big lump. She continues:

When you haven't got a waistline you are a big lump. I had to adjust to the fact that I didn't have a figure any more. I considered that I used to be a reasonably smart dresser, but I don't feel that really dramatic, sharp, bright sort of thing is so good when you are sitting in a chair. So my dressing changed dramatically; I became pretty and softer.

Frances speaks of the importance of another person affirming the reality of her 'new body'. The reactions of a new partner enabled Frances to incorporate her damaged bodily parts into a new, on-going self-image. She says:

I had real feelings of inadequacy, it was all tied up with my feeling of not being happy with my body. He was able to talk about my body in total terms. In talking about the parts of me that worked and the parts of me that didn't work he would say things like he loved me because of this and that and also the parts of you that you don't think work so well. So for me it was really important to have someone accept me as I was now and to affirm that I was still a person that was worthwhile and lovable, and it didn't matter if my body was different. So it was important for me in accepting my body as well.

Sally is a very successful wheelchair sportsperson. She has developed big shoulders by playing sport, and because of what she describes as 'my masculine ways—my tomboyish ways, my roughness on the basketball court', she now feels the need to appear 'more feminine'. She says: 'The thing that people notice about me is my hair now. I am described as that girl in the chair with the long hair, or you know, Sally with the long hair. Most guys compliment me on my hair. I am lucky it is nice.' Tina claims that she does not always like the way she looks now: 'I don't like the look of my body when I look in a full-length mirror. I prefer to see myself with clothes on, I don't feel happy without clothes.' At this point in our conversation Tina reached behind her to open a wardrobe which revealed a wonderfully diverse collection of beautiful clothes.

It is clear that clothing is a very important tool of re-embodiment. Both the women and the men acknowledged the importance of clothes selection, especially now that many of the other avenues of 'impression management' are no longer available to them. Alison says: 'People in institutions look disgustingly unfeminine. I don't think that I ever did, but I know that a lot of my peers did when I was there. I couldn't get over the way their parents would just dress them in really daggy clothing.' Alison claims: 'You must become very conscious of what makes you look good and what makes you look bad.' Robyn resented the boots and the strong, lace-up shoes that she had to wear when she was younger, and particularly her inability to wear high-heeled shoes during adolescence. Rosemary claims that television and magazine images of attractive, sexy, feminine women 'don't really matter to me. I am who I am, I can't change that at all.' The necessity of wearing an ileostomy bag around her waist means that Rosemary is restricted in her choice of clothes to those without a waistband. She wears mainly pants with an elastic waist with a shirt over the top: 'I only wear dresses occasionally, skirts and dresses tend to be hard to manage when I need to empty my ileostomy bag.'

Sally says that it is very hard to buy clothes for herself now:

> *I tend to make a lot of things. Because I have some feeling, I find sitting in jeans most uncomfortable, so I just won't wear them. I am more comfortable wearing lycra pants. That's just me—lycra pants and an oversized T-shirt, or something like that. Now, more than ever though, I have a need to be feminine, so I buy blouses, but I tend to buy things that have a batwing to de-emphasise my shoulders.*

Pam, whose accident happened many years ago, feels that she has come to grips with her appearance:

> *I know how I can dress and how I can't. Again I am lucky in the sense that I can afford to buy nice materials. But I still have to make them, and that can frustrate me because I see beautiful clothes, Diana Fries for example, and I love them but I can't wear dresses at all.*

Just as Pam craves a particular style of dress that she can no longer wear, Tina has a fantasy about the kind of clothes she would love to wear: 'I would like to wear a black leather, or a red leather one-piece dress, with a plunging neckline and a very tight skirt, and oh, high-heeled shoes. My mother would disown me!' Although Tina goes on to say: 'I have been trying to analyse why I am like this', it is not hard to imagine why someone who has spent a large part of her life in an institution, and has had to depend on others to fulfil her bodily needs, may crave to display herself in such a way. That she has been able to retain such a spirited sense of self in spite of the pragmatism of her experiences is a major personal triumph.

Wasted leg muscles are often an issue for the men and women who have experienced spinal injuries. Bob says: 'Being such a low break I don't get spasms so I have very skinny legs. I have been told, mainly by ladies, that I look better in baggier pants. Tight pants don't look good. I guess I am aiming at looking the closest I can to the way I looked before.' George, on the contrary, feels that he has become less concerned with some of the details of appearance management since his accident:

I think that I have become less vain. I used to be very particular, I used to floss my teeth and trim my nails and that sort of thing. Now I am not able to do a lot of those things. I probably feel a better person for it. I used to waste too much time on trivial things. Because I can't be fussy it's better, you do what you have to do.

George explains how his dressing has changed since his accident several years ago: 'I dress more like a crip. I wear more comfortable clothing, more practical clothing—stuff that is easy to get on and easy to move around in. I wear stuff that I can put on myself. I don't wear shirts with buttons because it means that someone must button them for me. So I wear shirts I can slip on and off, like windcheaters.'

Peter says: 'My appearance is important. I try to make sure that I appear as normal as possible, that I sit up straight, and that my wheelchair is one that people will comment on as an accessory, rather than an invalid chair. In my dress I try to maintain an appearance so that people will think that I am just a normal person sitting there in a wheelchair.' Peter suggests that as a twenty-six-year-old man with a disability, he is taking much more care to create a conventional appearance of masculinity than he would have done if he had remained a twenty-six-year-old able-bodied man: 'I feel that I was always careful about my appearance, whereas now I am super careful. It is very important to come across well to other people.'

Ian talked earlier about the way he constructs his external appearance to conform to the appearance of people in similar work positions. At home, on the other hand, Ian has 'no problems wearing shorts and things like that around the home or where I'm not somewhere where I'm trying to make some sort of impression'. It is not Ian's leg wasting that worries him as much as the lack of muscular control in his abdomen: 'I now have a huge stomach, and there are no muscles to hold that in—and of course I have a depressed chest and arms which look like I'd been in Belsen.' When I commented to Ian that he appeared to have very square shoulders and sat very straight in his chair he replied:

Well, I have always worn a surgical brace from the day all this started. Medical people tell me that it is quite ridiculous. I actually had people discouraging me from wearing it, but I've always done it. I have a very slight scoliosis which I think would have been worse without the brace. But it also supports

my stomach, which otherwise is incredibly uncomfortable. I get
enormous wind if I go without it. After I have it on I actually
can breathe better too.

Appearance and body image are integral to embodiment. While
attention to the exterior surface of the body occupies us all, concern
with the hair, clothing and other dimensions of appearance takes on
new importance in the project of remaking the body after visible
bodily disruption. While re-embodiment may defer to conventional
representations of masculine or feminine appearance, evidence of
inventive, richer, less-confining projects points to more optimistic
possibilities for these and other bodies in the future.

3 Social routines and relationships

Intimate relationships are the essence of everyday social life. We are social beings: we interconnect and relate together in pairs and in groups, at parties, assemblies and convocations. Friendships, companionships, romantic relationships, marriage and parenting bring richness to the routines of our daily lives. Birth, marriage, divorce and death are events of great social importance because the traditions and continuities created by marital, parental and filial relationships fill our lives with meaning and purpose.

Self-identity is constructed through social relationships. We learn who we are and our place in the world through our relationships with others. Friends, lovers, family, and more distant associates reflect us back to ourselves. They complete the person's self-image in a manner that can be only partially fulfilled by the person himself or herself. It is the body, however, that is central to face-to-face interaction. It is the body that enables the individual to participate in social encounters, the body that engages in and alters the flow of everyday life. The body is critical to the development and maintenance of social routines and relationships.

The work of Erving Goffman has demonstrated the centrality of the body in the development and maintenance of social encounters and in mediating the relationship between one's self-identity and one's social identity. The body is a resource which is managed in a variety of ways in order to construct a particular version of the self. Although Goffman's explorations of the body in *The Presentation of Self in Everyday Life* (1959), *Behaviour in Public Places* (1963)

51

and *Stigma: Notes on the Management of Spoiled Identity* (1964)
were published well over a quarter of a century ago, the influence
of this scholarship remains alive today, in particular in Giddens's
recent study of the reflexive constitution of self (1991).
Although the body is the focus of attention in Goffman's explorations of everyday interactions, this body is not autonomous, but is
encumbered by 'body idiom', or 'conventionalised discourse'
(Goffman 1963, p. 34). Body idiom comprises 'bodily appearance and
personal acts: dress, bearing, movement and position, sound level,
physical gestures such as waving or saluting, facial decorations, and
broad emotional expression' (Goffman 1963, p. 33). While amenable
to individual intervention, these activities are not completely control-
lable by the individual, and for this reason they act as a constraint
within which body management occurs (Goffman 1963, p. 35). Thus,
for Goffman, the body has a dual location. Although the body is the
property of the individual, the body is defined as significant and
meaningful by society (Shilling 1993, p. 82), by sources located
outside the body which are largely out of reach of those people who
are the subjects of their influence. Although Goffman went further
than most in considering the nature of human embodiment in
interaction (Turner 1992, p. 44), in his work we still learn less about
the body than we learn about the receptiveness of the mind to shared
vocabularies of meaning (Shilling 1993, p. 88).

Giddens's recent works on intimacy and self-identity (1991; 1992)
are heavily influenced by Goffman, as is his earlier work on modernity (1990) (Manning 1992, pp. 179–83). The essence of Giddens's
work is the dialectical relationship between the personal and the
social; changes to intimate aspects of personal life are directly tied
to the establishment of wide-ranging social connections. By exploring
innovative social forms, people develop coherent and continually
revised biographical narratives (Giddens 1991, pp. 54–5) in an active
project of reflexive reconstruction of the self. Although Giddens
professes the importance of the body to modern lifestyle (1991), his
body appears more as a thinking, choosing agent, not as a feeling,
being agent (Turner 1992, p. 87). Giddens's predisposition towards
the rational body may replicate some of the problems inherent in
Goffman's work. While appealing to the insights of both Goffman
and Giddens, this study directs attention to the phenomenological
body as the core around which a more satisfactory self can be
reconstructed. Through the interweaving of their phenomenological
bodies and social categories people work actively on their own
re-embodiment.

Relationships are conducted within frameworks of taken-
forgranted behaviour and expectations. Social imperatives pattern
interactions and limit the possibility of dissonance. By controlling

the factors that enable others to evaluate us, we attempt to manage the situation in order to produce the most satisfactory outcome. Etiquette, manners, politeness and 'proper behaviour' facilitate social relationships and minimise the likelihood of factors that might disrupt the situation (Elias 1978).

The visibility of bodies (Goffman 1964, p. 64) enables people to make assumptions on the basis of the body that they see, and provides little protection for the individual from the evaluations of others. The body idioms that people use to classify others, however, are also used to classify the self. If the appearance or movement of a person's body allows others to judge that person as a 'failed' member of society, the person will internalise that label; this will be reflected in a sense of 'spoiled' identity (Goffman 1964). It is not hard to see how the body mediates the relationship between social identity and self-identity, and how bodies may disrupt social relationships. Because the 'stigmatised' individual shares beliefs about the body and its performance with others, these beliefs may dictate the individual's self-image (Goffman 1964, p. 17).

Just as the body is critical to social relationships, unsatisfactory relationships threaten embodiment. Relationships are critical to the development of the embodied self, but they can also be a dangerous site of disembodiment. Identity is shaped through sociability, and social interactions of all kinds—from transient to long-standing, from intimate to impersonal—have the potential to enhance or diminish self-identity. With so much at stake, it is clear that social relationships are a source of potential concern for people with damaged bodies, and for us all.

The people in this study have experienced profound change to their visible bodies, but although this damage has disrupted their embodied selves, it has not annihilated them. These people still possess and occupy their bodies. Though damaged, their bodies remain a conspicuous force in social encounters and an integral component of social action. Identities can be moulded or remade in social interaction. It is the obduracy of embodiment that directs the processes involved in remaking the body.

Goffman's work on stigma, failed people and spoiled identity (1964) is important, but overestimates the power of social classifications and may underestimate the corporeal component of action. Although the people in this study have experienced the disruptive power of social categories within social interaction, they also demonstrate the powerful and creative ways that they use their bodies in the on-going process of re-embodiment. It is through embodiment that social interactions are reshaped and reforged after serious disruption, and the body is central to this process.

SOCIAL INTERACTIONS AND RELATIONSHIPS

How have the men and women in this study used their bodies to manage the disruptive components of social intercourse in order to preserve old connections or discover new interrelationships which will enhance, not damage, their embodied selves?

Although Sally feels frustrated about the fact that she is not able to mingle in crowds, she is well aware that there are many issues beyond the physical attributes of the chair that restrict sociability. She says: 'I know that there are a lot of people who have a lot of problems with sexuality, but I guess I have more of a problem getting people to accept you to start with.'

The visibility of a damaged body increases the vulnerability of a person to the scrutiny and appraisal of others. Although bodily appearance may be a difficult issue for all women, the women in this study have fewer resources to employ, and fewer alternatives to pursue, in protecting their bodies from the assumptions of others. As Sally says:

In a chair you are seen so much more easily. Compared with a guy in a chair, he can do anything—he can be radical, he can be in a family, he can be out on the town doing anything. But a woman in a chair, that's a bit funny, that should not happen. It is a very outmoded way of thinking, but I do notice it, and many people have discussed it with me.

Sally has observed the experiences of her friends in wheelchairs over many years. She says:

There are a lot more women out there who are prepared to overlook the chair and go out with a guy in a chair than there are men who will go out with a woman. It seems to me that men want a woman to be something to look at. When you look at a chair people are not going to be sort of, oh wow!—they would rather a tall blonde with long legs. They don't want a girl in a chair. They see her as a crip. Whereas girls don't feel the need to have this tall, good-looking guy next to them—they go for the guy himself. So I think that in terms of initially meeting people, women in chairs have much more difficulty than guys in chairs.

Sally's anger at such blatant expressions of the double standards of gender is obvious: 'The discrimination of being in a chair is enough without the discrimination of being a woman.' She goes on:

This is the frustration that I feel. I've been in social situations where I've been out of my chair sitting—I always tend to sit in the pub chairs or whatever—and I was with my girlfriend who is a tall blonde with long legs who attracts guys like nobody's business. I was sitting there on this particular night when these guys came up to talk with us, they were really relaxed with us and everything. We all decided to move on to another place as a group. She (Sally's girlfriend) got up and got my chair for me, and I sat in the chair. The guys' faces just dropped, they couldn't believe it. The rest of the night they were asking her questions about me, and she was saying, 'Ask her, don't ask me. Ask her about herself'. That was it, that was really it!

Jenny, too, talks of the power of the disordered body to disrupt social interaction. She remembers:

People stopping me in the street and telling me that if I believed in Jesus I would walk again. I remember going to a supermarket with Bill—I was buying some tampons—I handed over the money and they handed the package and the money back to him! Even when I was working at (names the place)—I'd been to a meeting with the Minister on a professional issue and as I was coming back into the building someone told me that if I pressed the button the lift would come!

The idea that a physical disability simultaneously renders a person intellectually disabled is a common experience for many of the informants in this study. That visible change to one part of the body can disenfranchise the person from competent participation in all avenues of life is a prevalent and destructive assumption. The notion that belief in God could restore a damaged body blames the victim for his or her own condition, for choosing not to walk again. The continuous impact of such covert factors in routine social interaction perpetuates the disembodiment of people with visible bodily change. Jenny goes on:

You've got a whole context of people that are defining you in a particular, subnormal way, and defining you in a non-sexual way. But I refused to believe that because I was a paraplegic my life should be any different. I knew that there were limitations on what I could do, but it did not seem to me that I should change my thought processes about my life.

Yet despite her resolve Jenny had the clear message that some men saw her as damaged goods, an experience shared by many of the other women informants. The logical extension of this pejorative perception is that you should be grateful for any attention that comes your way. Jenny talks of the beginning overtures of a relationship with a man who was a health professional:

> *He wanted to have a more sexual, long-term relationship. What was interesting was that he was quite angry and got quite nasty that I wasn't grateful for the relationship. I know some women with disabilities talk about men who choose them because they've got disabilities. I actually think that he was, in part, attracted to me because he thought he had the capacity to dominate. I mean it's almost like a wife in a violent relationship. There are some men who choose to be with women who have disabilities because they are less threatening and because they could be more domi-nant. That certainly did not suit my personality or my feminist beliefs and all of that.*

The condition that caused James's paralysis was obvious from the time he reached eighteen months of age, many years ago now. Although relatively independent until the age of fifteen, James required progressively more assistance from his parents to do the routine tasks of body maintenance. In his twenties he went to the city to live in a rehabilitation unit in order to acquire equipment, especially an electric wheelchair, so that his body would be less onerous for his parents to manage. The rehabilitation unit repre-sented the first time that James was in the position to relate with people other than members of the family. Recalling this time, James says: 'I am very aware when I look back that I was like a man who just stepped on to the moon. To me it was really stepping into life.'

Ron says: 'Not very many people ever bother to get to know Ron the person. They see Ron in a wheelchair and that's it. They don't see Ron the person. I give a lot of myself to my friends and to my family.' Ron echoes the frustrations experienced by many of the other informants in this study at the restricted views that people may have of men and women who live in and with visibly different bodies. He says: 'That's why there haven't been relationships, I think people see me in a wheelchair and they don't see beyond that.'

In the case of Sally, the act of transferring from a bar chair to a wheelchair, it seemed, transformed her from potential partner to a 'crip' in a chair—from an active participant in heterosexual sociability to a person who could not speak for herself. Personhood, womanhood, cognition and intellect collapsed in the act of transfer. Although Sally's visible body had initiated the interaction and her conversational style had been sufficient to sustain it, all evidence of normal womanliness disappeared in the face of the overriding category of 'crip in a wheelchair'. While men in wheelchairs enjoy many of the benefits of men in general, it seems that women in wheelchairs are doubly disadvantaged. If able-bodied women are seen as trespassers in public space, then women with disabilities are not only 'out of place' in relation to gender but also 'out of place' in relation to their dominant category, 'cripple'. As 'cripples', patients and invalids—as depersonalised, disembodied, passive, powerless and degendered people—women belong in particular places, not the real world of able-bodied men. How can women with damaged bodies transcend such discrimination?

Mary's experiences reinforce many of Sally's contentions. Mary's husband was killed in the accident that caused her permanent paralysis. Mary says: 'It is different when you go out into company. I was in the position of being not only in a wheelchair, but also being a widow.' Mary explains: 'As a widow you are not quite as bad as a separated or a divorced single parent, but you are still a liability to your friends because you are the odd one out. If you come along, are you making eyes at my husband?' The dominant model of coupled sociability constructs single status as a dangerous category. Singleness continuously threatens to disrupt the norm of coupled heterosexuality. Exclusion may be the easiest way of dealing with this danger.

Yet, paradoxically, Mary says: 'Being in a wheelchair helped me because they looked at me differently—as though, she couldn't possibly!' A male friend from (names country) told Mary of the comments a colleague made to him when he was leaving for a holiday in South Australia: ' "Oh, going to see your widow friend are you?" Ha, Ha, Ha, nudge, nudge, wink, wink. Another colleague said, "Oh don't be silly—she's in a chair" '. Mary added, 'End of issue!' Mary suggests that being in a wheelchair may have facilitated her inclusion in sociable contexts again. Her damaged body rendered her 'safe' in terms of gendered sociability. Her inclusion in social life as a single woman was won on the grounds of her disembodiment. Her bodily alterations were seen to cancel out her sexual desirability. Her paralysed body made her less womanly. At this price, however, her inclusion was too costly.

Although a large body of literature points to the double burden of disability and womanhood (Browne et al. 1985; Campling 1981; Deegan & Brooks 1985; Dovey & Gaffram 1987; Fine & Asch 1988; Lonsdale 1990; Morris 1989), Ruth suggests that being a woman may have made life with a disability easier for her. Ruth says: 'It is more acceptable for a female not to be physically active than it probably would have been for me to have said that had I been a man.' Ruth suggests though, that while it may be more acceptable for a woman to appear weak, to be physically inactive, she must

look as though she can care for others. A man may display his
physical strength and gallantry by helping a woman, yet the woman
must look as though she can reciprocate the favour by emotionally
caring for a man.

Tina has spent most of her life in residential institutions of one
kind or another. She says:

> I had one person I stayed with in an institution who had the
> mentality of maybe a two or three year old. I learned how to
> cope with it and how to communicate with her. The most
> important reason why I stayed with her was because she couldn't
> go around and talk about my life. I was able to keep my privacy
> because she wasn't able to talk about it. Had I been with someone
> else they would have been asking me what I was doing. I really
> got shitty having to tell everyone in the institution what I was
> doing.

Tina's privacy was guaranteed by the limited intelligence of her
room-mate. In return, her room-mate received Tina's support and
companionship. The pragmatic nature of this reciprocal relationship
served both women's needs.

The attitudes of others may be formidable barriers to the social
reintegration of people with damaged bodies, but practical issues
associated with mobility and access present another range of problems.

Ian considers that lack of spontaneity is one of the most serious
impediments to the development of interpersonal relationships for
people with damaged bodies. Ian says:

> When you're in a chair you often get locked in a room. If you
> are in a group of people you can't actually join in the conversa-
> tion easily. I have a lot of difficulty hearing. You're down lower
> and when people talk in the circle the only way you can do that
> is to sort of push in and quite often when you do that other
> people get pushed out and so the circle gets broken up. People
> get to one end of the room and you can't get to them because
> of the furniture, or whatever. And if you go to a party or
> something you tend to get stuck in a corner and it's about the
> people who come and talk to you rather than those you might
> wish to go and talk to.

Ian goes on: 'I think that this can lead to other things, one being
that you may become a bit overly sensitive sometimes and for some
people you might even appear a little cold and separate from them.'

Describing a wedding he attended Ian says:

> *When we got there the owner of the premises came out and said to my wife, 'Are you bringing him in?' She said, 'No, I usually tie him up to the front door-post, would he be all right here?' as quick as lightning. If you were a bit thin-skinned you might never go out again. People would say fairly amazing things, never talk to you and assume that you were just this thing, and look quite askance at the fact that you were going to come in and muck up their nice little arrangement.*

Mary says: 'I always found it difficult to join a group of people. I preferred to listen and ask questions. On two legs you can wander from group to group with cups of tea or plates of food, or just quietly find a group and listen in.' Pam, too, claims that she is frustrated when she 'can't do the traditional hostess bit of handing food and drinks around and moving around amongst people, and cleaning up after entertaining'. Sally claims that she 'found it really difficult to talk to people before my accident. If someone said hello to me I would hardly say hello back, simply because I was not confident in myself.' Sally continues: 'Before the accident I could get away with it (poor verbal communication) with body language, but afterwards, in the chair, you are restricted. You suddenly have to sit up front. You realise that people are going to be looking at you. You can't just hide in the shadows in the corner, people see you.'

A damaged body confronts aspects of gendered sociability, and alters aspects of social interaction. Mary says that now she must continually bear the burden of responsibility in social contexts. She says:

> *I always have to make the first move. People look at you and you can tell that they are not sure that if you don't work from there down, do you work from there up? You have to be prepared to bowl up and say hello. If you are a woman in a wheelchair your footplates and your feet arrive first, then your knees. By this time all the members of a group have stood back in order to include you, and they all have to look down at you. This is all a real interruption. So they decide to resume the conversation, but they are aware that they must include the wheelchair down there. You have to be prepared to do much more than your share, you have to convey the message that I am here and it is alright to speak to me, and you have to learn to ask questions in order to get involved in the conversation.*

Sally confirms many of Mary's points:

> *If I am at a party it is very hard to mingle if you are in a chair.*
> *For a start, you are at the level of other people's waists so you*
> *get a crooked neck looking up at them. If you are looking at*
> *someone eye-to-eye you can hold their attention; sitting down*
> *there it is very difficult. Last Saturday night I was at a party*
> *where there were 70 to 80 people in a fairly small area. I knew*
> *a lot of people around the room, but I could not communicate*
> *with them unless they came to me. People have to choose to*
> *come to see me.*

Bridget claims that the worst aspect of her bodily crisis is the
disruption her body causes to her expectations of teenage sociability:
'I can't walk and be with friends from school, or with friends my
same age. I can't do the things that people my age do—go out with
boyfriends or in a group.' Unlike Bridget, Jenny, through her work
is involved in interpersonal analysis and remediation. Yet she too
felt deeply upset by the disordered interactional patterns produced
by her bodily changes. Jenny says: 'I soon learned that I had to
direct people what to do. What's difficult about that is that you've
got to have the skills and perception to do that. I'd just do things
that would establish me into something different from the stereotype,
and I used non-verbal behaviour to do it.'
Peter says:

> *I can recall that before I was in a wheelchair I would have gone*
> *across the street to avoid someone in a wheelchair because I*
> *didn't know how to approach them. If they should say something,*
> *what would I say back? Remembering what I was like, I feel*
> *that other people are probably the same. For that reason I try*
> *and overcome this discomfort for them. I am the one who asks*
> *the questions or who says 'hello' first to make them feel at ease.*

Ron claims that meeting people and developing friendships has
been extremely difficult since his bodily catastrophe. He says: 'All
the people that I know have been associated with the care side of
my disability. I am not a person that goes to pubs. Because I'm
dependent on people you can't just spontaneously go out and sit in
a bar and drink.' Although Ron has found it extremely difficult to
develop personal relationships of all kinds since his accident, he is
currently in a relationship. He talks about his new friend:

> *She is more than my girlfriend, she is a really good friend. We*
> *both talk about a lot of things in the future to do with what it*

would be like for her being not so much the carer, because there are systems available that are in place for that, but I am always conscious of how much she does and how much work she would have to do. She is quite happy to put me to bed and to do those things that have to be done. But I'm very conscious of her not working too much, of not asking her to do too much because it's important to me that she doesn't feel that she's got to do everything.

Ron says that the most difficult aspect of intimate relationships is his inability to be spontaneous, to be able to do spontaneous things: 'to be able to gently touch someone, to be able to make the person feel good'.

George's greatest fears associated with personal relationships are related to his loss of bowel and bladder function. He says: 'I'm still sorting these things out. As you progress more, you get more confident. Once you are in control of everything [bladder and bowel] yourself, things change.' At the time of the accident, George explains, he was 'in a transition period where I had left school friends behind and was making work friends. It's a bit of a lonely space. It's a transition period for everyone.' George says that his social life is beginning to develop a little now, some three years after the accident.

Although Anthony had been in an 'extended relationship' for some time before his accident, he claims that it was many years before he felt comfortable with his sexuality again. He says: 'It was the one thing I pushed away—relationships. I had a visitor from a local town where I used to come from at one stage. She was studying up here. She used to pop down and see me and used to make sexual advances to me. But I couldn't respond—I didn't want to respond. I pushed her away. I wasn't ready.' Like many of the informants, Anthony considered that bladder and bowel dysfunction constituted the most disruptive imped-iment to the development of relationships and, indeed, to the establishment of friendships in general. Anthony says:

> *For the first seven years I wore a condom and external drainage. I found that really affected me, it really affected my sexuality. It affected my ideas about my body and my sexuality. I found that really difficult. You have to feel comfortable with yourself—not knowing when you are urinating is very scary and very threat-ening. You feel that people must be very conscious of it. For this reason, you don't put yourself in a situation where that might happen.*

Bob claims that it was 'about four years' after he left the unit before he began to feel comfortable about himself again. He says: 'I learned about myself partly by myself and partly from people, just normal, everyday meeting people in the world, going out. I learned to pick up signs to recognise that there might be a lady attracted to me and to learn to do something about it.'

David's disembodiment occurred when he was fifteen years old. Because David's paraplegia is incomplete his bowel function is undisturbed and he can participate in penile/vaginal sexual intercourse. About five years after his accident, David married a woman who was a registered nurse. In discussing intimate relationships David says: 'I've always been a reasonably confident person but I've always had a nagging doubt in the back of my mind—why would you want to go out with someone like me?'. David claims that his marriage broke up because he continued to have relationships with other women. He says: 'I just can't leave women alone.' Elaborating on this statement David says:

> *It might be a bloody excuse, but I still think there's some foundation in it —I was fifteen when I had my accident. I had just lost my virginity and I was at the height of my supposed sexual pinnacle. I had missed it right from fifteen to eighteen. I probably was not aware of my sexuality until I met my wife. I gradually found my sexuality again with her but I was keen to try out all sorts of things, not just extra-marital affairs, but things like threesomes, all sorts of stuff. I just went mad. I attribute that to the fact that I missed out on everything. My wife was willing to experiment, that is until she got pregnant and had our son.*

Ken suggests that women with damaged bodies find relationships harder than men in similar circumstances. He explains: 'I think that body image, and this is chauvinistic but that is the way of the world, seems to be significantly more important from a male perspective towards females. Men place higher value and priority on physical appearance than women do.' Ken goes on:

> *As for me—I could never contemplate being married to a paraplegic. That's as simple as I can put it. And yet I have no problem perceiving an able-bodied person being married to me. Males still think very much in stereotypes and I think they are much more susceptible to that than women are. I think that women are much more flexible than men in that respect. So from my experience I'd say that the majority of men seem to be in relationships and the majority of women don't.*

After the breakdown of Mark's marriage a woman relative assumed the role of carer. Mark says:

I had an elder sister who was my mother figure in many ways when I was a young kid because my mother had been ill at the time I was born. My elder sister had played a significant role in my upbringing and lo and behold, here I was again in a childlike state being dependent and needing somebody to take care of me and look after me.

Mark says:

This was an ideal role for her and she used to say sometimes when people asked her what she did, 'I look after my paraplegic brother'—which I didn't like very much.

Mark claims that his re-embodiment was facilitated by his second relationship. He says: 'That was a really important part of my second relationship. My partner woke up in the morning and would say, "Good morning" to my legs and that was a really important part of my integrating my body, accepting my real body.' Mark's second partner was able to acknowledge Mark's body rather than disattending to it as Mark himself had been encouraged to do after his accident. Mark goes on:

I suppose with men it's not really OK to talk about your feelings and to express your feelings. That carries through the whole rehabilitation process. We must deny that we are feeling sad or angry and we aren't in any way given permission to talk about those things or to feel OK about those things. It's almost as if you have to go out and do something physical, but don't get into this feeling stuff because you'll become morose.

Former patterns of sociability and relationships are disrupted by a damaged body. Bridget says:

Some people came to see me from [the country town]. *They felt sorry for me. Some really did not know what to do. A girl who was in the car came and saw me in hospital, but she didn't see me very often. The driver was sorry for what she had done, but she didn't want to give away much. She got married last year at Christmas, and has a boy. She got married in* [country town] *and she did not even invite me. I guess she was embarrassed. Push me under the carpet, wipe her hands clean. I really don't have many friends now, particularly young friends.*

Joy describes herself before her accident as 'wild, not rebellious, just a wild young girl who never had any problems attracting people—who never had problems getting boyfriends. I was never without a boyfriend: I always had somebody, whereas now it is different—I am months and months without a boyfriend.' Discussing male friendships now, Joy says: 'There are too many arseholes. Too many men see me in a chair, and they say "Yeah, I like her"—but they won't go out with me. It's all right for them to come and have sex with me, but they won't take me out anywhere—they find that too hard to cope with.'

In identifying the difficulties they have encountered in developing heterosexual relationships, the women in this study are unequivocal that men with similarly damaged bodies face far fewer difficulties. Tina says:

> This is because women are usually seen as the carers. It is very rare to find a man with the same qualities. I do know that there are men out there with a nurturing nature, but it's more unusual than usual. It's been portrayed on television that a woman with a disability is like lead around someone's neck, a burden for a man. But I've got attendant carers to help me get up and do all of those things. Men don't realise that a lot of women in wheelchairs are independent in most ways, but you don't get an opportunity to explain this.

Despite the wide range of difficulties associated with heterosexual relationships reported by many of the women, some women recounted more facilitative experiences. Sally says:

> I guess I've been lucky with the people I have chosen or who have chosen me. The man I went out with for two years until I broke it off two years ago was a good example. He was so easygoing with the chair and with me as a disabled person. He said, 'Well, I guess I don't really see the chair'. Now that is a unique person! You've got to see the chair first, but he did not see anything other than me.

Although Ruth has always enjoyed satisfactory relationships with men, she does not feel dependent on a partner for her survival. Ruth credits her introduction to feminism as an adult student with helping her to make sense of the world. She says: 'Feminism has also given me a fantastic network of women friends whom I call on regularly. Perhaps I am short-sighted or too optimistic, but my theory is that whatever happens I will cope. It's simply a matter of coming up with the strategy for working out how you're going to do it.'

Like Ruth, Tina enrolled in a women's studies course. Tina claims that this was 'quite an eye-opener' for her 'because I suppose I had been kept very ignorant. I had never thought of things in that way. Sometimes I don't even think of myself as a woman. In fact, most of the time I don't really think of myself as a woman. I just think of myself as me—not as a man, or a woman—just sort of me.'

Mary claims that it was about three years after the accident before she 'began to feel attractive again'. She described two particular men 'who treated me as an attractive woman; it was nice to feel that way again.' Mary says: 'I suppose my sexual awakening had occurred or something, because my brother and father mentioned one day that I looked very attractive—so that made me feel good about myself.' Speaking of her own second marriage, Mary says: 'Well he took me on as I am. He knows what it is all about.'

Jenny also talks about a 'sexual turning point'—a time when she felt she could accept herself, and feel acceptable as a sexual partner again.

I went to this conference and I felt this wonderful, magnetic attraction—this sort of sparkle for this man. I didn't tell him that I had worries sexually—and we had this very glorious sexual relationship for about a year. I obviously behaved differently after that because within weeks I'd had various other married men whom I was working with proposition me. I was projecting something, and I think that maybe, I was using my body differently as well.

Frances, too, speaks of the importance, but also of the terror involved, in exploring new relationships—the juxtaposition of danger and opportunity. She says:

My changed body image had been enormous. But displaying myself in a new sexual relationship has been pretty terrifying. The first real sort of sexual relationship I had with someone after my marriage broke up was in fact with a man I had been very close to previously. He had been aware of me as a sexual being before that but very much in the context of being a very physical person. So to take up that relationship again was very scary. I was very lucky in that he had always been a very caring man and so he dealt with it [her damaged body] very well. It was my fear that was the terrible part. I had real feelings of lack of spontaneity in the sexual relationship, and feelings of inadequacy. These things were all tied up with my feeling of not being happy with my body. I think one of the most important things to me during that relationship was the fact that he could talk to me about my body in total terms.

Frances reports that her

> *husband hadn't been able to see me this way because he wanted*
> *me to be better. Giving into the fact that I was going to remain*
> *this way was a denial of me. But in that process we lost something*
> *because we were still clinging to that past rather than trying to*
> *move on and saying, 'OK, this is now'. So, for me, it was really*
> *important to have someone* [a new friend] *accept me as I was now*
> *and to affirm that I was still really a person that was worthwhile*
> *and lovable and it didn't matter if my body was different. So it*
> *was important for me in accepting my body as well.*

Alister has always had a very close relationship with his wife.
She visited him every day during his long stay, some eight months,
in the rehabilitation unit. As Alister says: 'With two young sons
about one and two years old, it must have been very hard on her.
It used to take her about forty minutes to drive from where we lived
to the hospital. It wouldn't have been easy on her.' Now, many years
since the accident, Alister says of his wife:

> *I would classify her as my best friend. I know that she does a*
> *lot for me, but I know I play a part as much as she plays a part.*
> *She gets me up in the mornings and gets me on my way, but I*
> *know that I fulfil a role within the family in that I provide an*
> *income and I provide a positive atmosphere within the family*
> *unit as much as she does.*

Ian has been married twice; his first marriage lasted for eleven
years. Ian claims that:

> *The main problems with marriage with someone with profound*
> *disabilities such as I have is the problem of showing affection. You*
> *can't move. You can't make 'thing of the moment' gestures to*
> *people. Impulsiveness is something you can't engage in. It's very*
> *hard to reach out to somebody and, because you're protecting your*
> *independence a lot you tend to get a bit of a hard exterior. You are*
> *aware most of the time that there's an area of discomfort around*
> *you and you have to ignore these things. And you ignore things*
> *over so many years that you tend to get a little bit tougher about*
> *emotive things. I think that some of these things are a big problem*
> *sometimes in marriages. But the other thing is just not being able*
> *to do things—impulsive things—as you would like to do them.*
> *You're clumsy, you're unable to do them. Well, I mean, in*
> *lovemaking situations you perhaps don't have as many adaptive*
> *alternatives as other people have. You lose spontaneity.*

Robyn claims that she 'wasn't marriage material' because of her life-long disability: 'I had a lot of boyfriends but when they got serious I would say, "I don't think marriage is for me".' Despite these expectations of herself, at the age of thirty Robyn married a man with a disability, though one different from her own. Talking of the reactions of her family and friends to her marriage, Robyn says: 'Some had the holy horrors. How dare I! Oh goodness me—you can't get married, you are a disabled woman. What if you have children? How will you manage?'

Even though Pam's ten-year marriage survived the vicissitudes of her damaged body, Pam is unequivocal that her accident changed her husband's life. She says: 'I always knew that I had his one hundred per cent support—I never doubted that, and he never gave me cause to.' Pam is clear in attributing her successful rehabilitation to social factors. She says: 'I came from a social level that was educated enough to be able to understand and accept what had happened, and my friends did not back off and not know how to cope.' Acceptance and understanding, though, are not just intellectual capacities. Social class, and its component elements such as occupation, residence, income, association and access greatly facilitate people's ability to 'accept' and 'understand' physical loss, and are thus extremely significant facilitators of re-embodiment. Sally comes from the same social class background as Pam, and the fact that she received compensation for her accident has enabled her to explore interesting areas of life, something that has been extremely influential in reconstituting her embodied self. Although she acknowledges that marriage and motherhood are potentially important aspects of her embodiment, she feels that she would not grieve if she did not marry, that she could transcend these categories.

Joy feels more strongly than Sally about these central tenets of emphasised femininity. They are central to Joy's ideas about her own embodiment. She says:

> I want to be a bride one day and I want to be a mother one day. You know, I want to wear a wedding gown and stand up in a standing frame while I am getting married and wear that dress. I have a dress here—a beautiful, long lace black dress that I haven't worn since my accident. I'd give anything to wear it again, walk around in it, stand up in it.

PARENTING

Parenting a child may be the most significant activity in many people's lives, bringing pleasure and satisfaction as well as pain.

Child rearing is also a powerful vehicle of social reproduction; values, attitudes and world views are perpetuated by this means. Ideas about the capacities and limitations of men's and women's bodies are internalised, enacted and rewarded within the institution of parenting. Motherhood is still seen as a critical feature of womanhood (Oakley 1981; 1986), yet aspects of this activity may be detrimental for many women. It is not principally the physical experience of child bearing that is damaging to women, but rather the institution of motherhood under patriarchy (Rowland 1988, p. 133). The 'social cult of maternity' (Edgar 1980, p. 433) and the 'concept of childhood' (Summers 1975, p. 166) are keystones of the nuclear family. The cult of maternity expects a certain type of maternal body, one with particular physical dimensions and shapes and a degree of physical fitness and competence (Matthews 1984, p. 175). The good maternal body produces a good child.

Pregnancy, labour and lactation are bodily activities. Motherhood, in addition, is a complex social construction that has come to embrace diverse elements. It is the conflation of child rearing with child bearing under patriarchy that has been so detrimental to women's choices and possibilities. Motherhood has expanded to incorporate a wide range of household tasks, all of which are heavily enmeshed in moral meanings and value (Cass 1987, p. 181). How have the women in this study remade their embodied selves in terms of these strong social imperatives?

Despite overcoming her own expectations of marriage in relation to her damaged body, Robyn persisted in her reservations about motherhood. She said to her husband-to-be: 'We will get married on the condition that there is no family.' In fact Robyn had a child, a daughter. She says:

> I wanted to do the best for my child, so while I was in hospital I had a tubal ligation. I suppose I expected that as a woman I had the role of homemaker, and my expectations were very high. I wanted to achieve to prove that I was like everyone else. I was very houseproud then. I was very involved with the needs of my family.

Rosemary became much more assertive in discussing the possibility that she may be unable to fulfil aspects of the traditional gender division of labour within the household because of the restrictions of her body. She says: 'Well, I see it like this. I don't see a woman as having to be barefoot in the kitchen and pregnant.' She continues: 'And as far as cleaning up everyone else's messes, well—if they make a mess then they should do it themselves anyway.'

Alison claims that her sexual identity is challenged not by her paralysed body, but by the fact that she is unable to have children. Years of involuntary contraception during her time in institutions has made pregnancy difficult, if not impossible, yet Alison still sees motherhood as a crucial aspect of her womanhood.

A major reason for the breakup of Jenny's relationship after her accident was the issue of children. She recalls that 'one of the first things I asked about was whether or not I'd be able to have children. After that was cleared up, I was concerned about how I would be able to lift a baby up off the floor, or how I would put it to bed.' Jenny sought the advice from a woman with a similar physical loss who had several children. 'She said "I don't bathe the baby nearly as much as other mothers would—I do this but I certainly don't worry about that—you'll be fine" '. Jenny has subsequently had two children, the experience of 'which has been very pleasurable and I don't think it's a difficulty for the children'. However Jenny says:

People often ask me whether the children are mine. Even with a newborn baby people would say, 'Oh what a lovely baby! Is he yours?' I think that we will always get stared at in any circumstances, but when I was pregnant and would walk down the street [in a wheelchair] *with the other baby I would get stared at all the time.*

In the cult of maternity a woman with a damaged body, it seems, cannot also be a mother. New life cannot issue from such a body. If it is assumed that the body is unable to perform the obligatory mothering rituals required by our society, then it follows that the woman should not bear a child. If able-bodied women find themselves caught in the gendered conflation of child bearing with child rearing, then women with damaged bodies are doubly disadvantaged since they not only share the implications of this illogical association, but must also wrestle with their status as damaged beings.

Frances had three children at the time of her body crisis. Although her husband was keen that they have more children as they had planned, Frances was adamant that they did not. Frances said:

It was very clear that I could no longer have my role as a woman dependent on my mothering. I had entered a new phase in my life, whereas my husband was very keen to continue the focus of parenting in our lives. I couldn't handle parenting being the focus of our lives because I couldn't do it as well as I used to.

Joy is unequivocal about her desire to have children. She says:

Having a child is very important to my femininity. But I don't want to have children until I am about thirty. And I just hope I've got a good man to help me along with it. Before I would have never thought twice about bringing up a child by myself, now it's not possible, it's not possible at all. I'd have to have someone with me all the time to help me do it.

Bridget is more phlegmatic. She says: 'If I found the right man I would really love to have a kid, but I am not ready yet.'

Rosemary, too, is clear about her desire to have children. She says: 'Every now and again I see a little brat, and I think "No, I am not having kids", but, yeah, I would like a kid some day.' Rosemary can foresee some practical difficulties 'in changing him or her, or things like that', but 'the issue hasn't come up yet, so I haven't talked about it with doctors or with anyone else'. Although Rosemary claims she would like to have a child, she doesn't see motherhood as a critical aspect of her womanhood.

The possibility of inherited transmission complicated Ruth's decision to have a child. Ruth says:

I never doubted that I would be able to look after the child. I knew it would be hard, but I had lots of support. The issue of caring would never have stopped me. But I looked at the quality of my life and I decided that my life was bloody good, that I was damned pleased with it. So that's helped me make my decision to have a child of my own.

If I had chosen not to have a child solely on the basis of maybe not having a perfect child, that would have been very damaging to me because that would have been damning myself.

Frances did not experience the full impact of her disrupted embodiment until she returned home after an extended period of time in a rehabilitation unit. She says:

Even though I had had a great deal of contact with my children right throughout the hospital period, I found that particularly my one-and-a-half-year-old child had a lot of difficulty relating to me. It was quite terrifying for him to be left home alone with me. There I was sitting in a wheelchair not able to pick him up. He would frequently run to the front of the house where we had all glass doors and scream out for his father. It was almost like he was imprisoned with this person he didn't know. I felt his real sense of fear that if anything happened I couldn't do anything about it. So that reinforced my feelings of absolute hopelessness. I wasn't able to change his nappies or do anything like that. I felt quite inadequate about that.

Mary's youngest child was five months old at the time of her accident, so although the baby was not injured, she shared many aspects of her mother's rehabilitation. Mary's older two children were cared for by different relatives, and although Mary regrets that she missed so much of the older children's growing up, her continuing close mothering relationship with the young baby was extremely important to her. 'Having Ann with me kept me going—she was very important to me, and I think that I was important to her.' Several friends breast-fed the baby until she joined Mary in the hospital on about the third or fourth day after the accident. Mary continues:

I don't think I would have survived as well as I did without Ann. I still wanted to feel wanted. That's why I appreciated Ann so much because she of all my children would come and cuddle me. The others would come and cuddle, but they cuddled me because, 'There is Mum, say hello to Mum'. So what do you do—you give Mum a cuddle. They didn't need me the way I wanted to be needed.

Emotional closeness and a sense of being needed by others were critical components of Mary's re-embodiment. The continuity of mothering in Mary's life was a powerful connection with the values and priorities of the everyday world during nearly two years of hospital and institutional living. This socially sanctioned identity may well have protected her from slipping into the world of patienthood, a destination where many informants found themselves, at least for a time (Seymour 1989, chs 6, 7).

Frances talks about what she saw as the

problem-solving type of rehabilitation. Obviously part of the rehabilitation process was to get me home and that was clearly a view of me going back as a mother; but it was very much an occupational therapy model of how I was going to manage stairs and how I was going to get to and from the bathroom. But never how was I going to manage to look after my baby. So there was always this split, they never quite got it together, they could always deal just so far with the problem but not the stage that was really going to impact on me. I was going to find ways of getting around from one place to another myself, but where I really needed some guidance was how the hell I was going to cope with the fact that I really didn't feel a mother to my baby any more. How was I going to deal with that?

While the attitudes and the practices of some health professionals may have restricted her re-embodiment, Frances claims that her children also, unwittingly, exacerbated the impact of her bodily disorder. Children's experiences of ill health are usually optimistic. In the early stages Frances's children were able to regard her as a patient who would get better. Frances said:

As they got older and were starting school they started looking around a lot more and defining people in categories of who was able to do things and who wasn't. So, for a while, I became a person in the category of a person who could not do things. I found that hard to deal with. It would come through in their drawings and in their expectations of what I could and what I could not do.

Mothering is still an important component of Mary's life. She describes her feelings when she first learned to drive a car with hand controls several years after the accident. She says:

I remember coming home one day from doing some reading in my daughter's class at school. My mother had called in and I had not been home. She couldn't even get in because the house was locked. She didn't know where I was—this was a nice feeling that my parents who had been doing so much for me, and my father who had to do all the driving for me, just did not have a clue where I was. I had been out, and they did not know where I was! Suddenly I gained independence!

Mary compares this experience with the joy that adolescents must feel the first time they go out without prior negotiation with their parents. 'Now I could do things. Other people did not have to drive my children everywhere. I could be part of my children's lives.'

Although Pam had three small children at the time of her accident, the ability to have children was still an important issue. She says, 'I remember asking about my periods because they disappeared for six months, and the doctor said that it was just shock and that they would come back. At the same time he explained to me about the fact that I could still have children.' Pam's husband commented that he felt 'that if I became pregnant that it might be the straw that would break the camel's back'. Pam, on the other hand, said that the doctor's pronouncement was very important to her. She said: 'The comfort to me was that I certainly hadn't lost that capability. I think that is a very reassuring thing for a woman. In your own mind you are still capable of that most female function. I can remember thinking that meant that I wasn't so different after all.'

Like Mary, Pam describes the enormous significance of relearning to drive a car for people deprived of ambulation.

I know there were all sorts of limitations, that I just couldn't do lots of the things that other families could do. There was no way I could take them [the children] to the parklands or go for a walk in the hills, or take them to the beach and make sandcastles because I just couldn't get there. I used to compromise—I'd take them down to the beach, buy fish and chips and sit in the car and eat them. They were still too little for me to set them loose.

Men with spinal injuries may experience dramatic changes in fertility as well as in sexual practices. The changes experienced by men with these injuries may also have profound implications for the expectations of their wives or partners. Maintenance of relationships may involve intensive renegotiation, but the problems faced by people who are not involved in a relationship, or who have not had children, can be profound.

In discussing the issue of procreation Peter says: 'Knowing that I cannot have them [children] now, it would have been nice to know whether I had the ability to produce children.' Yet Peter claims that this fact 'hasn't devastated us at all. We found that we will live life differently, and make the most of it in a different way.'

Ron says that he would like to be a father. He knows that the chances that he can have a child are extremely slight, but he says: 'I would like to look into it'. George echoes Ron's words when he says: 'I guess I'm still fairly young, but I had a sex life that I miss. I really wanted to have kids.' Bob now has three children, a daughter in her early teenage years born to his partner at the time of his accident and two young children conceived later. The incomplete nature of Bob's spinal injury has preserved his fertility, unlike many of the men. Despite the fact that he has seen his teenage daughter only once in the intervening years, the issue of fatherhood has been very important for Bob. He claims that he feels 'a little bit sad that I don't get to see my daughter in Melbourne. I see my two children in Adelaide every second weekend and I have them on Wednesday nights. I get to see a lot of them, I think it is very important.'

Like Bob, David has an incomplete lesion, and he too has been able to father a child. David says: 'The reason I've got only one [child] is because I'm not married any more, otherwise we would have had some more.' David goes on: 'I was lucky that I could do it naturally. Lots of people are not so lucky. I have no regrets about having a child at all. I love having my son. He is a fantastic kid. It is fantastic being his dad. I love and enjoy the weekends I have with him.'

Discussing the issue of fertility, Ken says:

> *Well, it's important and it's not important. Grace and I would like to have a child between us but it's not something that is of critical importance to our life or to our relationship. I'll follow through with the program* [a fertility enhancement program] *and see how it goes, but if it's going to get to a point where it will be complicated or there'll be surgery involved, we're going to have to sit back and re-evaluate that. I'm not going to feel less of a man because I can't have a child.*

Mark claims that fatherhood was always very important for him; the implications of this particular loss concerned him from the earliest days of his bodily damage. He says: 'I was devastated about the end of the genetic line—no infinity—no on for ever and ever—this was it. My partner and I talked about IVF programs. With my first wife we talked about it and wondered about whether we should or what would happen.' Although Mark has never fathered a child, and his loss of fertility occurred more than twenty-five years ago it is clear that the issue is still important enough for him to recently consider going on the IVF program again. Mark says:

> *I think my* [new] *partner was more keen than I was. I could more or less take it or leave it. My partner was getting the message very strongly that you're not really a woman until you have had a child. In my first marriage the woman was just in the process of finishing off a relationship and the dynamics there were interesting in that the man was really put out, not so much by the fact that she was ending the relationship, but that she was ending the relationship to develop a relationship with me—a person in a wheelchair, a cripple, someone who is not a real man—and that was deadly stuff.*

Ian's extensive body damage was the result of an infection rather than spinal injury, so his fertility was not impaired. Ian has had four children, two with his first wife and two with his second wife. Ian says:

> *It has been extraordinarily interesting to observe the differences between my two experiences in parenting. In the case of my first*

wife—and if I say this I mean that there is blame on both sides—I took a very accepting role. The negativity of disability perhaps. Although I had a very aggressive business mind, on the home front I was probably much more accepting of a lesser position than I should have been. When my first two children started to go to school they were embarrassed about their father being in a wheelchair and they asked if I would never go near the school. Very stupidly, I agreed with that. My wife thought that this was a good idea too. And so they lived some sort of other lifestyle. That was a terrible mistake. And that affected my eldest son in particular very, very badly and, I think, to a lesser degree, my daughter. My wife and I broke up when they were around eight and nine years old.

EMOTIONAL AND PRACTICAL SUPPORT

Spontaneous expressions of emotional closeness are an important component of relationships. Discussing cuddling her grandchildren Pam says: 'They have all learned to climb up on my lap, to lean against the wheelchair and to push the wheelchair from the time they were walking. There doesn't seem to be any reticence about it. That's the way I am and I think that they have learned to cope with that.'

Jenny also discusses the issue of direct contact with children. The act of hugging or cuddling is obstructed not only by mechanical impedimenta, but also by loss of the ability to initiate spontaneous movement. This loss may be compounded by other people's difficulties in knowing how to react toward the person with a visibly different body. Jenny says:

It was really noticeable when I gave a conference presentation with a co-worker. There were people there who knew us both equally well, in fact some people there knew me more. These people came up after the presentation and gave Vanessa a hug, but they didn't give me a hug. I soon learned that what I had to do was to tell people to kneel down and give me a hug. What's difficult about that is that you've got to have the skills and the perception to do it.

The inability to spontaneously translate emotions into conventionally recognised acts of endearment can seriously distort personal interrelationships. Much is lost when you must direct someone how to hug you.

Ambivalence about the disordered body is compounded by the

reticence of others to react in an expected manner. Jenny talks of
her experiences with her partner on early visits home. 'I remember
him saying that he was scared to hug me, to touch me, in case I
broke. He was fearful about that, and also about my new body—and
I was fearful about his acceptance of the new state of my body.'
Jenny also talks of her feelings of alienation from her body during
her days in the rehabilitation unit.

*I can remember feeling that I needed to be touched. I remember
thinking that they should have masseurs attached to the unit
because of the physical deprivation and the degree of pain and
stress that your body is going through. Your body is handled,
but not touched. I remember thinking what I need is for someone
to be coming in and laying hands on me.*

Jenny differentiates 'handling' from 'being touched', and attributes the latter with reintegrative power.

Peter has always been close to his family and this closeness has
been especially important to him throughout the long process of
re-embodiment. As Peter says: 'If people are from the country, in
particular, it's very difficult because they have no support from family
and friends because of their isolation. People who don't have support
find it very difficult to get through. There's no one there telling them
that they're doing a good job, and there's no one there to come
home to.'

On discharge from the rehabilitation unit, Ron returned to the
country to live with members of his family. Ron's extensive bodily
damage necessitates constant dependency on others. Although he is
on good terms with his family, this arrangement was far from
satisfactory for everyone involved. He now shares a house in the city
with a younger sister. Although this arrangement has some problems,
it also has many advantages for both of them. His previous experiences with non-familial carers have been much less satisfactory.
Describing his move to the city from the country town, he says:

*It was OK initially sharing with people, but then they began to
intrude too much onto my life. And there were many unpleasant
experiences in my own house. I have been ripped off—people
have cleaned me out, moved out in the early hours of the
morning, cleaning me out of all my money. I found it difficult
to find responsible people. I have shared with some people that
have been good, but they would neglect to let me know that they
were going to be late. In my life there are things that you have
to do—like emptying my leg bag. It's just thoughtlessness, they're
just not thinking about these things.*

After a long stay in the rehabilitation unit, George returned to live in a flat on the side of his parents' house where his parents still cook and take care of him. Discussing his future plans he says: 'I think I will take the normal path that my brothers did and stay at home as long as I can. The record for that was age thirty, so I can relax for a bit.' Anthony, too, came from a large family. His memories of the early days after his accident at the age of eighteen were of being surrounded by people, lots of friends and family. 'My mother stayed there [the hospital] a lot of the time. That support for me was really important.' Bob's experiences of familial support were very different from those of Peter, Ron, George and Anthony. Although there were thirteen children in his natal family, Bob seldom saw members of his family during his time in the rehabilitation unit. Bob says: 'I was a bit angry about that but I worked out later that it was because they all found it [the accident] more difficult to come to terms with than I did.' Despite the fact that Ken had married and left his natal home long before the accident, the breakup of the relationship he was in at the time of the accident necessitated his return to his mother's home. David's youth (fifteen years old) made his return to live with his mother less problematic, but still extremely difficult for them both.

Joy's mother was very supportive. 'Mum was there from the second I woke up until the second I went to sleep every day for the first three weeks. Mum lived for me, she breathed for me.' Bridget's family lived in a country town some distance from the rehabilitation unit, but they too were 'over quite a lot of the time after the accident, they came in every day—they were very good to me'. Rosemary comes from a 'close-knit family'—she is well incorporated into their lives and relies on them for many practical and emotional aspects of her life. Pam says: 'The most important thing on my mind in those first years was learning to cope with my family. I just wanted to be back into my family life.' Mary, like Pam, had been married for some time and had a family of her own at the time of her accident, but she says of her natal family: 'We are a very close family, we still are, and we were then. We are very family-conscious; we are very interested in each other and our families.' Although Mary's baby lived with her in the rehabilitation unit, Mary's parents and siblings took over the responsibility of rearing the older children during the long period of rehabilitation. She says: 'I live near one of my brothers now. Our children—his children and mine—have had a lot of time together because of my circumstances.'

Yet despite the enormous amount of help that she has received from her natal family, Mary feels continual tension between the vulnerability of her body to breakdown and disorder and her role as a mother and carer of others. She talks about one particular

incident when she developed pressure sores on her sacrum for which
she was not able to seek proper medical attention because 'who was
going to look after my children?' In the end she became 'very ill
indeed, and ended up in hospital for a very long time'. This tension
has abated somewhat since Mary has remarried and her children are
now teenagers, but one senses she speaks with a conviction which
comes with experience when she says: 'Women are carers and men
are cared for'. Gender is the major predictor of who will care for
others. Women, rather than men, are the 'kin-keepers' (Braithwaite
1990, ch. 5).

Sally, too, has a very close and supportive natal family. She says:
'I had a lot of family support because there was a lot of understanding. Mum had a little trouble. She felt that perhaps "we had
to give up everything and look after Sally" '. Sally had already been
living away from home for two years, so 'coming back with a
disability and a different way of life, which I had to learn to live
with as well as my family, was very demanding and hard work for
everyone'. Sally says that the most difficult thing for her mother was
to curb 'her basic motherly instincts. I had to make her understand
that I will ask her when I need help: she had to learn just to let me
struggle, and to watch me do that.'

Ian has not been able to live by himself since his bodily catastrophe at about twenty years of age. He has received continuous
support from many women—from his mother, from his aunt who
was a retired nursing sister and who looked after him when he first
came out of the hospital, and from each of his two wives. Without
help, he says, I wouldn't survive one second. Ian's body is unable to
execute even the most basic task of routine bodily maintenance. He
is unable to get out of bed, dress himself or make a cup of tea. He
says: 'The drive that I've had to succeed has been because of me
thinking about the Home for Incurables as it was called in those
days waiting right over the back of my shoulder. And even today I
still recognise how close it is—it's only a day away from going into
one of those places.'

On the rare occasions that Ian has not been cared for by a woman
to whom he was related by family or intimate ties, he has had to
pay for personal care. Inevitably these carers have also been women.
Ian claims that he would much prefer to be looked after by a woman
than a male. When asked to explain his preference Ian says:

*I suppose it's the old sexual prejudice. I've often thought about
it. I'm very fussy who does that job. I can't stand the old matron
type. I'd much rather have anybody than those sorts, those
officious, bullying types of people. I'm not sure I can actually*

describe it all but it's, I think, a very male reaction towards that sort of domination.

James suggests that the patriarchal gender order is strongly implicated in the generation of different relationship expectations of men and women with damaged bodies, as it is elsewhere. He says:

[women] *always seem to have lower expectations from a marriage point of view than a man. Most men were seen as getting married. I think the motive was not because they were men being men, but as a way of solving their physical problems. Society saw women as being the logical way for him [men] to exist in society and unfortunately I think some fellows think that way. Those who think that way seem to be successful in finding someone. I'm beginning to think that I should think that way. Guys have said to me that life is so much easier when you're married.*

DEPENDENCE

The right to initiate activities with people of your choice, at a time that suits you, and in a manner that you feel you have chosen is the essence of freedom. Such freedom may well be an illusion of social governance, yet our socialisation manufactures the sense that our thoughts are our own; our defence of this notion continues to reproduce the idea of personal independence.

Abrogation of the idea of independence is a serious challenge to the embodied self. Dependency is the antithesis of personhood. To be dependent on professional workers may be costly enough; to have to rely on friends, relatives, children and partners may dramatically alter the delicate structures upon which such relationships are based. Relationships between people who are not formally related are often fragile: they may have been constructed on quixotic and unexamined affinities which may not stand up to change in the nature of the interactants. Obligations between legally related people—between parents and children, marital partners, or more distant kin—although more formal, may prove less substantial in practice. Relationships are fragile, delicate and vulnerable. Independence is highly valued, dependence is a costly state.

How do people whose bodies can no longer engage in many of the tasks of everyday life reconcile themselves to the changes this brings to a relationship? What losses does dependence incur? If friendships are constructed on the basis of reciprocity, can a friendship survive the accumulation of obligations incurred by a person who must continually rely on another? Can the self survive the necessity to substitute the actions of another person's body for the inadequacies of one's own? How have the people in this study experienced the impact of physical dependency on significant relationships in their lives?

The necessity to return to a dependent, parent–child situation in her parents' house which she had left two years earlier was a difficult situation for Sally, and similarly for many of the informants in this age group. Disembodiment compounds the vulnerability that often accompanies this passage to adulthood. The need to return on such inequitable terms is a difficult issue for many people with severe physical loss. 'Meeting a new boyfriend and starting to go out with him' was the catalyst for Sally to leave her parents' house, where she had lived for four years since her accident, and to live in a house by herself.

The death of a brother was the impetus for Alison to explore the possibilities of living outside the institution where she had lived for most of her life. She says:

> *Even though I had lived in an institution I had always depended on my family who lived in the country to care for me. My underlying thought was when Mum and Dad are gone, my brother will be there to look after me. Institutions are not so bad if you have somewhere to go on weekends or to get away from them with your family. I never had to strive for anything other than the security I had, and all of a sudden it was no longer there.*

This family tragedy was the catalyst for Alison to become a Christian and to live in a Christian community house. Alison says: 'The Pastor and the elders and their families opened their houses up and had these weird and wonderful people living with them—gangsters, prostitutes and people with wheelchairs. It was very interesting.' Alison found the new arrangements quite different from her previous experiences. She was no longer an invalid whom people were obliged to look after; she now had to relate to other people. She says: 'With the nurses you know they are getting paid, but my whole new way of life was that they valued me as a person, too. There was a whole lot of relearning of normal relationships that took place for me during this period, and that took a lot of time.'

The severity of Mary's injuries required her to stay in a rehabilitation unit for nearly two years after her accident. Relatives cared for her older two children while she was in hospital, and for a long time afterwards. Mary says:

> *My family was split up. I saw Alan once a month when my brother brought him over [from another State]. They had one*

small child, and my sister-in-law was pregnant. It disrupted their lives. In any accident you hear of the deaths, but you never hear what happens to those that survive. It affected not only my children, but it affected my parents and my brother and his family and many others besides.

Mary's sense of independence when she was able to drive a car again has already been documented earlier in this chapter. The car not only freed her from dependence on others, but it restored her freedom to initiate activities and to choose how and when such things would be done. Most importantly, it freed her from being continually on the receiving end of other people's generosity. No matter how altruistically motivated, such help places the recipient at severe disadvantage in terms of the informal rules of interpersonal relationships. Women, in particular, find this position difficult. A payment discharges the debt for professional services. Reciprocating the favour restores the balance of friendship or family relationships. For Mary, and many other women informants, the position of being the perpetual recipient of kindness and help from others with little hope of being able to repay these services filled her with an overwhelming sense of obligation.

Role socialisation prepares women for a lifetime of service to others; proof of duty well done is being 'needed' by others. The 'need to be needed' is a critical aspect of gender. Mary says:

My physical condition was such that I may or may not have lived. I did live, but for a very long time I very much wished that I had not. I could see no reason—my children were all dependent on other people. If they wanted something they turned to somebody else. They did not turn to me—I was totally dependent.

Frances shares much of Mary's anguish when she says:

At home my place had been taken by others. I learned that I had to become assertive again which is a skill I think I had lost in hospital. I had friends and family coming in to help, so I had to really renegotiate my relationships with those people as well as put myself back into the situation and prove my competence as a mother again. I had to learn to become quite strong again and say 'I am never going to get better if you keep on doing things for me'. And that was very hurtful to them because they had rallied around in a really crisis situation and their whole lives had been changed by this, they had changed. They had given up all sorts of other commitments to look after me. I was

criticised for being extremely independent, that I didn't know
how to accept help.

Although Pam needed less time than Mary and Frances in the
rehabilitation unit, she too was heavily dependent on women family
members to care for her three young children. My family—my
mother, mother-in-law, my aunty—rostered themselves to help while
I gradually learned to do things again. This took me about three
years. Although she shared Mary's feelings of dependency and obligation to others, Pam felt clear that this was the only way she would
be able to achieve the things she wanted to do in her life.

Although Bridget 'used to think that it would be easier to be a
paralysed man than a paralysed woman because men don't like to
look after women in wheelchairs', on consideration she thinks that
'women can take more mothering than a man—women are not as
scared to ask for help'. When talking about herself, however, Bridget
says that she feels lonely and is very depressed. 'It is a private
depression—something no one can help me with but myself.'

Although the social constructions of 'daughter' and 'son' also
involve many role expectations, increasing age renders many of the
assumptions ambivalent, if not obsolete. People in late adolescence
or early adulthood can be seen to be betwixt and between in terms
of their natal families and their adult lives. Because they do not fit
a clear social category, others may feel diffidence in approaching
them in social situations. An offer of practical assistance that may
lead on to an enduring friendship is much less possible in such
circumstances. Parental help may be resented because it is seen to
perpetuate the dependencies of childhood. Such liminal status may
offer limitless potential, but initially it may provoke the feelings of
rolelessness, anomie and alienation experienced by many of the
informants at this stage of their lives.

Although Joy is much in the same age group as Bridget, she feels
that she is in more control of these interpersonal dimensions because
she is clear about the importance of reciprocity in everyday life. She
says: 'I understand about returning a favour—anyway, I am a good
cook. So I say I'll help you do this. You do this for me and I'll do
this for you.'

If physical vulnerability can render relationships between grown
children and their parents problematic, how much more disruptive
must it be for a parent to have to rely on his or her children? Because
Mary has been susceptible to ulceration on weight-bearing parts of
her body, she has had to be very careful about inadvertently damaging these parts of the body that no longer have movement or
sensation. She says:

Alan, my adolescent son, had to help my also adolescent daughters to lift me soaking wet and stark naked from under the shower and on to my chair because I wasn't allowed to attempt this movement myself for fear of dragging on the newly healed pressure areas. You can never have any secrets from your children.

Mary suggests, though, that her dependence on her children for help in these intimate activities has had constructive consequences. Mary says that

I couldn't speak to my mother, and my mother couldn't speak to me about that sort of thing. I was determined that my daughters wouldn't be like I was. I've found that quite often a situation arises, and I'm quite happy to broach it and say, 'Do you know?' rather than waiting for them to ask me.

Necessity may have provided the opportunity to expand the narrow boundaries of intergenerational family relationships. In more usual circumstances, one's children, anxious enough about their own developing bodies, would be unlikely to confront their own mother's body in this way (Lawler 1991, p. 118). As Mary says: 'They've all seen me with nothing on, performing the most intimate—what's the word I am looking for—eliminations.'

Frances says:

For a long time the motherhood role was just not there for me, and I had to make very deliberate efforts to find things that I could do with my children. I felt I had no place in the house any more. I had all these friends who put the rubbish out, did the cleaning and everything, and all I could do was lie on a bean bag with people talking to me. I had a feeling of absolute indebtedness to my children. My three-year-old daughter used to empty my pans and that was something I felt dreadfully about. Here was me, I had done all those things for my children, and here I would watch my three-year-old child stagger up the stairs holding a bedpan, empty it and wash it out. I think my children have retained that sort of role of being responsible for me, particularly my eldest daughter who is now seventeen. The other thing was that they [her children] formed some very strong attachments to some of my friends. I feel that my children would often look forward to my friends coming far more than to my actual presence around the house. In hospital I had a place in the patient structure, but at home all my place had been taken by others.

FRIENDSHIPS

Mark talks about the importance of friends from outside the world of disability. He says:

> *I had a mate, a nice man, a wonderful man, a really good friend and he played a very significant role in my rehabilitation, he was a friend from outside, and he used to come in and visit and say, 'What are we going to do tonight, Mark?' and I'd say, 'Just stay here and watch a bit of television', and he'd say, 'Bullshit. We're going out.' And off we'd go out, and we'd go off to parties and all sorts of things. He really drew me out. He wouldn't allow me to sit about. He wanted to get on with living and he wanted me to be part of that and a lot of that was around parties and drinking, really heavy drinking.*

Although Ian's youth and the physical limitations of his damaged body precluded him from making extensive friendships with other patients while he was in the institution, he developed some important friendships during his long stay. Several nurses 'would go out of their way to see me and have a yarn'. Ian says: 'All of that, I think, was very important. They were great people.'

Mary pays tribute to her large natal family and the extensive network of connections that this generated. Initial formal associations, for example a sister-in-law's father, would lead to a chain of informal introductions far removed from the original connection. Mary says:

> *It became a bit of a saga. People would appear at my bedside and say, 'You don't know me but I know [names connection]'. People would often come initially for reasons like these. Eventually it dawned on me that they were coming because of me, not because they felt that they should come, but because of me as a person. And I thought, well, there must be something to living!*

Jenny's time in a rehabilitation unit was much shorter, and unlike Mary she sometimes felt quite overwhelmed by visitors. Jenny says there were people who had clearly decided that it was their duty to visit her. 'Such people were interrupting the work schedule that I was there to achieve.' Jenny resented these unsolicited visitors because her priorities concerned her rehabilitation, and spending time with people with whom she felt she had a closer relationship. The vulnerability of people with damaged bodies to the intentions and needs of others is often overlooked in the face of overriding assumptions about the neediness of these people for help. The motivations of people who 'give help' to others is seldom the subject of scrutiny. Giving assistance to others, whether professionally or informally, may help the donor more than the receiver.

Pam, too, talks about the difficulties of fitting visitors into the busy work schedule of rehabilitation. She says:

> *There were only a few people there* [in the rehabilitation unit] *that I had anything in common with. I certainly didn't develop any close relationships with other people while I was there. You see you are thrown into a very close situation where you are doing lots of things together. If your social or intellectual background is very different, then you only do what you have to do and you don't do any more. You virtually have to be self-sufficient.*

Pam's strong support from her family and past friendships enabled her to be 'self-sufficient' within the rehabilitation context—to escape immersion in the world of the patient (Seymour 1989).

Because Sally returned as a patient to the hospital in which she was employed, she found herself the centre of attention.

> *I mean it was lovely, but they had to stop the visitors because I was just not able to deal with it. It was just too many. I wasn't getting any sleep. But all of that stopped in a big way as soon as I went out to the rehabilitation unit because they weren't there to pop in. It was a bit devastating—all or nothing.*

Coping with people who were associated with the accident can be a difficult issue for many informants. Bridget's difficulties with this have already been mentioned. She says: 'Some people came to see me, and they felt sorry. Some really did not know what to do.' Not surprisingly embarrassment, sympathy, guilt and feelings of impotence overwhelm people's attempts to resume social relations after such a catastrophe. Bridget speaks of the difficulties people of her age have in meeting people. 'I really don't have many friends, particularly young friends—some people from church maybe. You can't go to pubs really, not by yourself, in a wheelchair you can't.'

Frances found that living overseas for two years a relatively short time after she left the hospital was very important in helping her to renegotiate the relationships with friends and family that had become so difficult for her during her sickness. Going away gave Frances an opportunity to review her life from a distance and, in particular, she said it made me really look at what my future was going to be, whereas back at home I had sort of looked at it very much as trying to regain the pattern of my past. Frances talks about making very strong and facilitative friendships when she was living overseas. She says: 'They had not known what I was so they were not trying to conserve the old me. They were very affirming. I suppose they were saying, "Fancy you travelling across the other side of the world with these three young babies". They were amazed at the way my children coped.' Clearly Frances was seen as exceptional amongst the people that she met in her new setting. She says:

> *It was very important for me to be seen in that way. It helped because I felt I was able to leave some stuff behind, some inadequacies, back in Australia. Here I was being regarded as a person who could really cope, whereas at home I was this person who couldn't cope, who used to be so and so and could do such and such, whereas in my new setting I was seen as quite an exception.*

Although much the same age as Bridget, Joy feels less inhibited by her wheelchair. When asked where she meets people now Joy replies: 'Oh, wherever. I just go and meet them. I go to friends' houses, or they come here. I meet them in town, or at a restaurant or pub. I like going to play pool at the local pub down here. It's great!' Joy says that she has a big group of friends, although few of them are women. 'My best friend is a man.'

Although Rosemary says that 'half of my friends have [names diagnostic category], the other half are able-bods.' Rosemary suggests, however, that she prefers to seek friendships amongst able-bodied people. She says: 'I've got a lot of very good disabled friends, so don't get me wrong. But invariably I find it easier to get along with my other friends. With my able-bodied friends I can talk about anything, and the medical side of my life doesn't have to come up at all.'

RELATIONSHIPS IN SETTINGS OF PROFESSIONAL CARE

The profile of the participants in a formal rehabilitation context is predominantly one of young, male clients and young female staff (Seymour 1989, pp. 62–3). A prevailing theme amongst the male informants was of relationships with carers in institutional settings. Peter says: 'For men, many relationships occur; these start with their carers, and this happens in the institution.' Peter attributes the high incidence of relationships that develop between men and their female professional carers to the particular problems the men experience with their bodies, specifically the problems associated with bowel and bladder dysfunction. He says: 'One easy way out of this difficulty is by starting relationships with nurses who understand these kinds of problems.' Initiating a relationship is extremely difficult since it often requires detailed explanation of bodily dysfunctions. Peter explains:

> *Once people are in a wheelchair, they are so much more behind the eight ball because if they were to begin a relationship it would require so much intimate explanation of their dysfunction to the other person who doesn't understand. When you meet someone for the first time, you try to strike up the relationship by talking about general things, like the weather and so forth—not about such intimate details of your body. What do you do? Do you tell them about your problem straight away and make them run, or do you tell them about these problems after you have got to know them and got to like them, and then they run?*

Anthony discusses the testing behaviours that frequently occur in this context. He says:

> *Some of the male patients would come out with fairly sexist sort of statements towards some of the female staff, often very openly. Sometimes they would set out to embarrass the female staff. It might have been a way for them to demonstrate power, when in fact many of them may have felt quite the opposite, quite powerless. It was a sort of joking behaviour, with heavy sexual innuendo—comments about the nurses' and the physiotherapists' bodies.*

Bob, too, discusses the masculine nature of the rehabilitation culture. He says:

> *Of course the patients are predominantly male, so that you're going to have masculine comments going on. A lot of the patients are between the ages of eighteen and twenty-five, a time when your masculinity is pretty important. It's a time when it is usual for young males to seek the people that they're going to marry, to seek relationships and the possibility of children.*

Bob claims that the women nursing staff were important in his re-embodiment. He says: 'I was still testing my own sexuality, my own sexual identity. I found it hard to distinguish whether the nursing staff were being nice to me, were being friendly, because they were nurses or whether they were being nice to me because they liked me.' Bob claims that he knew of many staff–patient relationships during his time in the rehabilitation institution. He says: 'They never really went on with me, probably because I was in a

relationship at the time. But since then I have seen lots of examples
of nursing staff matching up with patients.'

Anthony recalls relationships with some staff members of the
institution with great pleasure. He says:

> *In particular there was an older nurse there, Nurse X, she fitted
> into the role of 'mum'. She was the salt-of-the-earth type. She
> said what she felt, but would encourage and support people. She
> wouldn't put up with any nonsense though. Many of the younger
> guys who were in the unit respected her in lots of ways. I certainly
> did, she had a heart of gold.*

Although the physical impact of David's injury was immediately
obvious, it was at least two or three years later before he acknowledged the extent of his disembodiment. David says:

> *I thought I was fine for a while. I got a lot of attention from
> the nurses. I remember when I went home after being discharged
> from the spinal injury ward, I actually cried the first night because
> I didn't have my buzzer to call the nurse in. All I had was my
> poor old mum living way down at* (names outer suburb). *All very
> depressing.*

David's youth (fifteen years old) may have invested him with a
special status in the ward. David says:

> *I suppose I was a bit of a pet, and a bit of a brat—a bit of both.
> Some people adored me, and some thought I was a little pain. I
> had relationships with the nurses when I was in the unit. I was
> a pretty good talker. They were obviously a lot older than me,
> but I had some very interesting tête-à-têtes with the nurses. That
> got my confidence up.*

Nevertheless, David is curious about why these relationships
developed. He says: 'Maybe they wanted to associate with me
because I was something different, or maybe they felt they were
doing me a good thing.' Over the last four years David has had an
intimate relationship with a woman who works in a specialist
department of a rehabilitation unit. The two most significant relationships in David's life have been with women health professionals.

Gerald stayed at the rehabilitation unit at various times throughout his childhood in order to give his parents respite from their task
of caring for him. These occasions provided invaluable opportunities
for Gerald to learn more about his body. He claims:

It gave me a chance to meet up with a lot of young men who had become disabled over a period of time. We would go to drive-ins. I was a kid brother to a lot of them. I had lots of 'big brothers'. I would get lots of experiences from them. I remember one thing amongst many. One young guy, I guess he would have been about seventeen or eighteen, said to me 'It's really good fun undressing girls'. Since I didn't have any big brothers of my own this was important information.

Because of his youth Gerald, like David, was treated as a kid brother in the unit. It was here that he learned how to handle a wheelchair 'like a man'. He says:

The guys there were former bikies. They handled their wheelchairs quite differently to an older person. I wanted to emulate them. I needed these things. I needed to jump up and down steps and all the rest of it. When I got to [names another institution] they were horrified that I didn't wear a seat belt, that I would balance on my back wheels and whiz around. These things were really important to my independence. Clearly I was also learning about male culture.

Gerald, too, reaffirms the high incidence of staff–client relationships. He says: 'Yes, there was heaps of that. It was the same at the [names the agency where he spent a lot of his youth]. I had a very nice relationship with a sixteen-year-old nurse there when I was sixteen. I stayed there for about three months or so. It was strange when I look back at it, but it was lovely at the time.'

Many men attributed the preponderance of men who initially, at least, develop sexual or intimate relationships with health professionals to the perpetual anxiety people with these conditions feel about bowel and bladder continence. They suggested that it is easier to relate with a nurse, or at least with someone who is not so likely to be shocked by these 'uncivilised' aspects of their bodies. Ken, however, disagrees. He says: 'Well, I dispute that, I really think that's not right at all. I think the truth of the matter is the issue of access. Men have relationships with nurses because that's who they're in contact with, they're the people they see all the time and the opportunity is there.'

Mark claims that: 'There was a lot of what, in hindsight, could be seen as sexual harassment where the guys would try to grab the nurses on the breast or the bum or try and get a hug. What happened for me was a real sense of loss of my masculinity, my sexual identity. I was very aware that my sexual functioning had changed.' Although Mark devoted himself to sport as he was encouraged to do, he said

'I still kept thinking about sex and wanting to develop relationships. A lot of that then amounted to developing relationships with the nurses in the institution.' Mark claims that this was fairly common practice in the unit when he was there. He says:

> I used to have cuddles with the nurses in the morning and just as they were going off at night. I used to go to the drive-in picture theatres and to restaurants. I developed a very close relationship with a number of nurses there. One in particular, well two really, were significant relationships. Those relationships lasted for months and I was quite devastated over one when it broke up. It broke up because of my uncertainty about who I was and what I thought I was. These relationships were definitely sexual in nature.

Relationships of this nature, Mark claims, were pretty much routine for most of the young men undertaking rehabilitation at this time.

> These relationships were carried on with discretion, I think the nursing staff were told that you must be very careful about all this and, gee, the dynamics would be quite fascinating to explore—the sense of mothering, and caring that nurses get into and being confronted by young, healthy and to all intents and purposes, male patients.

Ian, also, claims that staff–patient relationships during his long stay in an institution were a critical factor in his re-embodiment. He says:

> Well, I'm a very visual person and some of those nurses, well it was a bit like the old game of show I suppose. I was always incredibly grateful to some of those girls. I never really understood what that was about or how, but a number would actually disrobe themselves to a degree and things like that, which for me was fantastic. This was terribly important—a fantastic piece of reaffirmation again, for some reason. The nurses of course were risking an amazing amount. I suppose it was in a very isolated area of the hospital, there was virtually no one anywhere particularly at night-time but even so they were risking an amazing amount.

Ian identifies relationships with other health professionals during his time in the hospital. These sexual and intimate relationships were extremely important to him. He says:

I think that some of these experiences that I had in that hospital were really the motivation to go on and to see that some sort of life is possible. I think that if I'd had a different attitude and none of that had happened in the early days, there might have been a very different outcome altogether.

Although obscured in terms of formal rehabilitative goals, intimacy clearly plays a critical role in re-embodiment. As Mark claims, it gives men a real sense of a way out. Less pragmatically, intimacy is the means by which new bodily pleasures and experiences are discovered, and the embodied self is revitalised. Intimacy is a crucial component of rehabilitation.

The body is central to the development and maintenance of everyday routines and relationships. Although a damaged body disrupts sociability and may disturb relationships, this chapter has highlighted the critical role played by the body in the restoration of the tasks and routines upon which everyday life depends. People may experience profound change to their bodies, but they still possess and occupy their bodies. They still have a body that enters into relationships with others, a body that may negotiate new understandings, a body that is capable of altering aspects of social reality. Although changed, the body remains a vivid, lived presence. Through everyday interrelationships with others the resilient body asserts its 'presence' and its 'aliveness' (Scarry 1985, p. 193). While bodily activities are conducted within a context of established social routines, the body may modify, alter or even transcend such social categories in the process of its own re-embodiment.

4 Sport and the body

In the midst of an exploration of appearance, relationships, intimacy, sexuality and fertility, a discussion on sport may appear out of place. The overall concept of rehabilitation used in this study relates to broad processes of re-embodiment, rather than to the more specific meaning of the term employed in medical contexts. However, strong narratives relating to athleticism and the physical body operate within this formal context. For this reason an examination of this aspect of the rehabilitation process is essential to understanding the processes involved in remaking the body.

The sociology of sport has been bedevilled with problems; it has been disdained by sociologists, and despised by sportspersons (Bourdieu 1988, p. 153). While the reluctance of athletes to talk about their activities is understandable, the lack of sociological interest in sport until recently is less easy to understand. It seems ironic that a topic that engages the body so directly and has such strong gender connotations should have eluded sociological attention for so long (Theberge 1991, p. 124). The reasons for this may be diverse, but the following factors may offer some explanation. The image of the physical body inevitably raises the issue of biological essentialism, a latent fear for sociologists anxious to escape associations with the biological body (Gilroy 1989, p. 166; Theberge 1991, p. 123). The seeming inevitability of men's biological predisposition (Hargreaves 1986, p. 142; Willis 1982, p. 117) may have deterred all but the most intrepid investigators. Involvement in sport and physical activity empowers men both physically and socially but has the opposite effect for women. Women who enhance their physical strength by weight-lifting or other activities often find themselves ostracised because of it (Gilroy 1989, p. 163). Sport seems so thoroughly masculinised that it is unlikely to be able to serve women's interests (Bryson 1987, p. 350; Inglis 1995, p. 6). Until recently gender has been seen as the prerogative of feminist theorising, resulting in a much less vigorous investigation of issues relating directly to men's bodies (Gilroy 1989, p. 167). The identification of sport with leisure or play has also served to deflect sociological attention from seeing sport as anything more than an activity that people pursued between other more important things, an issue of little significance in its own right (Bryson 1987, p. 349; Inglis 1995, p. 6).

Yet sport has been a key vehicle for the construction and reconstruction of masculine hegemony and for the power embedded in particular bodies. Not only does sport serve dominant interests by reinforcing the inferiority of women and their activities, but in supporting male bodily skills it sanctions aggression, force and violence as expressions of maleness (Bryson 1987, p. 349). It exalts hegemonic masculinity over other masculinities, a crucial factor in the continuing subordination of women (Cockburn 1990, pp. 82–3; Connell 1987, p. 85). The critical relationship between physical bodies and social power has been underestimated because of the association of sport with biology, maleness and leisure activities.

> Successful images require successful bodies, which have been trained, disciplined and orchestrated to enhance our personal value [. . .] The new ethic of managerial athleticism is thus the contemporary version of the Protestant ethic, but, fanned by the winds of consumerism, this ethic has become widespread throughout the class system as a lifestyle to be emulated. The commodified body has become the focus of a keep-fit industry, backed up by fibre diets, leisure centres, slimming manuals and outdoor sports (Turner 1984, p. 112).

Like appearance in relation to women, men's physical bodies are susceptible to the judgment of others, but this fact serves men in many other, more substantial, ways. Men's association with the physical body encourages them to think differently about their bodies and to use their bodies more powerfully in social situations. Patterns of behaviour and reaction that arise from men's long familiarity with the active, functioning body place men at an advantage in many other contexts. Although appearance and physicality both express the physical body, the implications are quite different for men and for women.

Bodily dimensions and strength are constructed and sustained by the contractions, strength and control of muscles and bones. Brain, spinal cord, nerves, muscle fibres, ligaments, tendons, bones and joints are evoked to create movement for the myriad functions and activities we demand of our bodies. Physical presence—the presentation of the body in space—is created by a similar synchronisation of bodily systems. Posture, shape, size, contour and dimension are as important to the body as its movements; a particular image of the male body becomes the ideal to which all male bodies should aspire (Connell 1987, p. 84; Hargreaves 1986, p. 170).

Gender socialisation encourages boys and girls to think about their bodies in different ways from a very early age (Gilbert & Taylor 1991). Girls are expected to care for their bodies. Demure attitudes, gentle games, polite behaviour, studied poses and graceful movements are valued in young girls. Anticipation of the rewards associated with feminine grace, beauty, fine movements and gentle demeanour in later life justifies the early and insidious instruction of girls in these attributes. Ballet classes, gymnastics, painting or elocution classes, music lessons or singing are persuasive agents of feminine socialisation.

Boys, by the same means, are encouraged in quite different behaviours. While girls learn to take care of their bodies, boys are encouraged to be careless with theirs. Although the rigid differentiation between boys and girls in the physical education curriculum of schools has been somewhat reduced, the social effect of the alleged biological differences will take much longer to eradicate (Hargreaves 1986, p. 176; Scraton 1987, pp. 160–86). Through rough and tumble and similar impetuous activities boys develop confidence in their bodies. Play involving running, jumping and fighting prepares boys to respond automatically to any situation. It is not surprising that most women lack confidence in these skills and that an increasing proportion of women seek to be trained in self-defence in later life, an activity that men take for granted.

Masculinity is expressed most powerfully in the physical body. Sport is a powerful institution through which male hegemony is constructed and reconstructed (Bryson 1987, p. 349). The sportsman is the product of many years of systematic training. Participation in team sports from an early age encourages boys to relate to others. The discipline of regular and vigorous training prepares the body for sport, but at the same time it inculcates values about working with others. Disregard for body discipline disqualifies a person from membership of the group for whom body discipline is the expectation for entry and a responsibility of team membership. Though some men may reject these values, for most men this early training becomes a life-long model of bodily action that has relevance far beyond the playing field (Connell 1987, p. 85).

Sport has been, and in most respects still is, a critical vehicle of gender. Sport is an important means by which boys develop ideas about their bodies that are significantly different from the ideas girls develop about their bodies. Parents, and later teachers, encourage certain behaviours, and discourage others (Bryson 1987, p. 358). Boys learn to see themselves in physical ways, to express themselves physically. Small wonder that many boys find sport and physical activities 'natural', at least initially (Willis 1982, p. 117). More importantly, boys learn to use their bodies in a way different from that learned by girls; these ideas become embodied. Ideas are translated into the body, both into its substance and into its movements (Connell 1987, p. 85). The relationship between boys' bodies and physical activity established at this early age will influence boys' confidence in their physical capacities as well as other people's expectations of them throughout their lives. Even men who eschew all associations with sport and exercise in later life cannot escape its early influence on their ideas about themselves and their bodies (Messner 1987, pp. 53, 65). Sport is not only a component of masculinity, it is also a critical force in the production and reproduction of the male body upon which masculinity is based (Hargreaves 1986, p. 176).

Yet sport is difficult for men. Only a minority of boys will develop excellence in athletics or other physical endeavours while they are at school, and far fewer will engage in these activities once their school days are over. Very few men will play team sports in the community. Although many men continue to play 'social' golf and tennis well into old age, many claim that their performances are often more destructive, than enhancing, to their self-esteem. Playing sport, then, is clearly an activity that is undertaken by a minority of men. Many men will enrol in gymnasiums or in fitness classes during their lives, while others will set themselves personal goals involving running, walking, bicycling or jogging. For most men, however, these activities will be no more than short-term enthusiasms motivated by current ideas about health or the risk factors of cardiac pathology. Playing formal sport, participating in athletic activities, or developing an enduring commitment to personal exercise programs are, in fact, minority preoccupations for most men.

Why, then, is there such discrepancy between men's enthusiasm for sport and their actual participation in physical activities? Thinking about sport, it seems, is more important than playing it. Interest in sport facilitates entry into male culture. Connections between men are forged by simply knowing about sport. Knowledge about the subtleties of scoring, about records and times of sporting heroes of the past, about the form and capacity of particular players, enables men to come together in a manner that transcends other, more structural barriers. Non-participatory involvement in sport—

watching sport, reading about sport, talking about sport, knowing about sport—is a critical element of masculinity, and a potent instrument of patriarchy. Connections between men engendered by vicarious involvement in sport are critical to male solidarity. However, sport plays an even more fundamental role in men's lives. Ideas of a successful sportsman are associated with particular bodily presentations and characteristics associated with strength, control, reliability, aggression, tenacity, discipline and competence. It is these ideas, epitomised in sport, and internalised by men because of their close association with sport throughout their lives, that influence the way men think about their bodies. These strong representations encourage men to think about their bodies in ways that affect other activities in their lives that may bear no relationship to sport, or indeed to physical activity at all (Hargreaves 1986). Few men are athletic, yet key values associated with athleticism correlate to the social construction of masculinity and permeate the bodies of all men. Detached from their original source, such bodily presentations are seen as natural attributes of men (Connell 1987, p. 85). Successful outcomes reinforce the social power of such bodily attributes, and reconfirm the legitimacy of a particular form of the male body. Bodily attitudes and actions arising from the 'game', the 'tournament', the 'fixture', the 'match', the 'event' and the 'competition' are transformed into patterns of bodily behaviour considered normal for boys and men in the playground, on the shop floor, in the boardroom and within the family.

Ideas of physicality inform the presentation of the male body in contexts where physical strength, size and aggression are frankly not required, but the dominance of the male body is also established by other characteristics related to sport. Team play prepares men for success in organisational contexts (Madison 1994). Familiarity with competition as well as co-operation, with tenacity and timing, with resilience and endurance, with quick response and with long-term strategic planning, serves men well in social situations. Decision making, assertiveness, 'seeing the bigger picture', defining priorities, identifying options, clear thinking, the ability to bring issues to resolution, all are qualities supposedly associated with men in committee rooms, on boards and in organisations (Madison 1994). Not only do such characteristics determine the relationships of power in these situations, but successful outcomes lead participants to conclude that 'men are better at these sorts of things', to see such attributes as natural to all men. The preferencing of the physical body in men's lives prepares men to perform in many other aspects of their lives.

Recognition of the potency of men's physicality in these situations and of the effectiveness of masculine styles of interaction leads many women to attempt to emulate the outward bodily attributes and presentations that seem to be so successful for men. 'Executive' or 'power' dressing—heavily shoulder-padded jackets and dramatically tailored, neutral-toned business suits worn by women in the 1980s— was an attempt to present women's bodies in a manner that conformed to the bodily presentations of successful male executives. Such strategies, though, are little more than mimicry, since men's association with physicality and the continual cultural reproduction of this connection have influenced men's bodies, and the way others relate to men's bodies, throughout their lives. Action, spontaneity, aggression, strength, confidence—key values of masculinity—are embedded in men's bodies. Women's attempts to copy the outward expressions of men's bodies will fail, since such imitation ignores the profound and embodied nature of physicality in men's bodies. Men's bodies have embedded these ideas; but within patriarchy, women's bodies never can.

The preceding exploration of key aspects of the ideology of sport has established the social context within which rehabilitation proceeds. Ideas of athleticism permeate the rehabilitative context and influence the practices involved in the work of reconstructing the body. The production of an athletic body represents the pinnacle of rehabilitative success. Although the overall concept of rehabilitation employed in this study relates to broad processes of re-embodiment rather than to the more usual and specific association of the term with medicine or the rehabilitation industry (Albrecht 1992, p. 28), this chapter will focus directly on the formal rehabilitative context in order to examine how powerful social narratives related to athleticism and the physical body operate in this context. This focus may seem contradictory, but neglect of this aspect of the formal rehabilitation process would represent a serious opacity in understanding the processes involved in remaking the body.

PHYSICAL CONNECTIONS

Twenty-three of the twenty-four informants have spent time in formal institutions and most of the men and women have spent a considerable time in contexts that exemplify the issues raised in this chapter. The overwhelming predominance of young men as recipients of spinal injuries rehabilitation services (Seymour 1989, p. 62), the physical nature of the development of spinal injuries rehabilitation (Seymour 1989, p. 56), the frailty of damaged bodies, and the context of crisis and uncertainty that envelops such profound bodily disruption contribute to the development of a rehabilitation project that is constructed around a physical/sport/masculine model of rehabilitation. While this model may be expedient for some men, other men as well as most women may be disadvantaged by this orientation. Although the focus on sport in physical rehabilitation correlates with key values associated with the physical body in the everyday world, this association may be a serious impediment to re-embodiment. This chapter will explore the impact of the ideology of sport on the process of remaking the body.

Not all of the twelve men and twelve women in this study have suffered spinal injuries. Medical conditions accounted for the extensive bodily paralysis of six of the women. Only two of the women were driving the cars involved in the accident that disabled them, while two other women were passengers in cars driven by others. One woman was knocked off her bicycle by a car driven by a drunken man, and another suffered injuries during house renovations. In contrast, only three of the men suffered from medical conditions, five were severely injured in motor vehicle accidents, one was involved in an accident on a motorbike, and the remaining three were injured while participating in vigorous physical activities.

Spinal injuries happen to young men. Of course women also injure their spinal cord, as this study clearly demonstrates, but the incidence of spinal cord injury is overwhelmingly higher in men than in women (Seymour 1989, p. 63). This dramatic fact cannot be explained by any difference in the strength or structure of the male or female spinal cord. Clearly factors that lead to injury of this vital part of the body must be examined in order to explain the high incidence of men with these conditions. What is it about the activities that men do that predisposes them to spinal injuries?

Men's work on building sites, on the land and in defence activities greatly increases the susceptibility of the male body to these injuries. Women's work seldom exposes the spinal cord to this type of danger. Men and women may not only work in different spaces, but they are also likely to behave differently in the same space. The epidemiology of spinal injuries suggests that although men and women drive cars, men drive cars differently from women. Men and women enjoy water activities, but men dive into shallow water while women swim. Rugby League and Australian Rules football need not involve greater speed or contact than netball or softball, but men's attitudes to their bodies and the manner in which they approach the game are vastly different from the way women relate to their bodies and to their sport. Such attitudes transform the game. Do men rush in where women fear to tread (Scraton 1987)? Courting danger, taking risks, defying the odds, testing the limits are critical to masculinity. Injuries resulting from this behaviour are clearly related to gender. Spinal injuries, in particular, are a masculinist issue.

The gender disparity in the incidence of spinal injuries is not reflected in the intentional selection of equal numbers of men and women to contribute to this study, yet gender is clearly a factor in the causation of these injuries. The discussion that began this chapter established the dominance of the ideology of sport; it seems likely that the issue of physicality is implicated in both the causation of spinal injuries in men and in the rehabilitation of these men. Such evidence from a small study like this is, of course, not conclusive. The particulars of the accidents that caused the injuries are largely lost in time and in many cases litigation; all remain enveloped in some degree of pain and grief. Even this cursory information, however, indicates that of the twelve women, only three were actively involved in factors that led to their injuries whereas nine men could be seen to be active participants in their own, 'accidental', injuries. This evidence substantiates the claim that men and women not only participate in different activities, but also approach such activities differently. It may well be that the physical characteristics of masculinity that led to the injuries also offer men their best rehabilitative potential.

PREVIOUS INVOLVEMENT IN SPORT

Many of the male informants had substantial previous involvement in sport and physical activities. Although Alister and his two brothers all played football at league level, Alister says: 'My father used to have a few kicks with us and muck around a bit in our younger days, but there was not a lot of football talk at home.' Although the lack of football-centred conversation in Alister's home seems surprising, Alister's subsequent statements may explain this. Alister was an 'aggressive player, and although other people seem to identify with someone who is a bit rougher', his parents found such conspicuous play harder to accept. Alister claims that his parents were not particularly proud of his sporting achievements; nor did they attend the matches in which he played. 'They used to when we were younger, but as we got older I didn't have a good reputation within league football. They used to get into too many fights trying to defend me so they found it easier to stay home.'

Anthony, also, 'was very good at sport. I played a lot of tennis and a lot of football. I got a great deal of enjoyment out of sport. When you are involved in sport to the extent that you are doing a lot of training, it is also your social outlet.' Bob, too, was 'very physically oriented' before his accident: 'I loved sport—football, table tennis, squash. I had a friend who had a houseboat. We would go down the river skiing.' Although George played football at school he did not make the top team, and 'never took it seriously'.

Nevertheless he considered himself 'a fairly athletic, fairly outdoors kind of person. I liked water sports—windsurfing, waterskiing'. Most weekends were spent staying in a beach house owned by his parents where he spent the days windsurfing and waterskiing and going to barbecues or to the local hotel to hear a band at night. Unlike Alister who was injured while playing his favourite sport, Anthony, Bob and George were injured while driving cars or motorbikes.

Ken was also very involved in water sport. Although he says that he was 'a better than average surfer', he claims that he was 'just a recreational surfer—certainly not competition standard'. He followed the surf, spending extended periods of time in well-known surfing locations in Australia and America. Speaking about the residential unit in which he lived at the time of the accident Ken says:

It was a great unit, it really was. It was next-door to a pub, 100 metres from where I worked and 200 metres from the beach so that I could look out of the lounge-room window to see what the surf was like. Most mornings I would get up at daybreak and have a quick look to see what the surf was like. If it was any good I would go and have a surf before work, and if it wasn't I'd go back to bed and get up later.

Ken was injured when he 'missed a corner and drove my car over a cliff'.

Ron's life before his diving accident was typical of the life of young boys in country towns in the mid-1970s. He left school at fifteen, four years before the accident. 'I wasn't interested in the school at all. I wasn't interested in the system, or the system was not interested in me.' Although he was engaged in hard manual work on a vineyard in his home town, he was looking forward to travelling north, finding work when he needed it for the next few years. Ron saw himself as a 'country boy', and as 'one of the boys' before his accident. This involved partying, drinking, plenty of camping and bike riding. 'We all had cars and bikes, and played lots of sport.' Ron played football, tennis, badminton and cricket.

Peter describes his life before his accident as a 'very physical, very active, outdoors life'. Although he lived in an outer suburban area of an Australian city, Peter's occupation at the time of the accident, and his job expectation for the rest of his life at this stage, involved riding horses. A bolting horse, in fact, was the cause of his serious spinal injury.

David, who describes himself as having been a 'young, loonish fifteen year old without much direction' was still at school at the time of the motor vehicular accident that caused his paraplegia. After a nine-month rehabilitation program, he returned to school, 'but half-way through my matric year it really started hitting me about my disability. I just copped out, and spent a couple of years doing nothing.' He was about eighteen before the full impact of his disability became apparent to him.

Unlike David, whose injury occurred in mid-adolescence, Gerald suffered severe bodily paralysis at seven years of age. Most people either are born with a disability or acquire it in late adolescence or in early adulthood. Gerald considers that 'I had the best of both worlds in that I had gone through to the age of six without any illness so I developed competent social skills along the lines of any other able-bodied child'. In early adolescence, membership of a scout group for boys with disabilities enhanced Gerald's sense of competence. 'We would often cook our own lunch on a fire that we had to light ourselves. This was the only opportunity we had to do something like this. We had to pitch our tents which meant hopping out of our wheelchairs and rolling on the ground. It was often great fun.' Gerald considered that the medical condition that caused his severe paralysis

> *happened early enough that I was able to accept my disability and come to terms with it in a way that an adolescent male would find more difficult. I grew up with my wheelchair in the same way that I guess other guys would grow up with blond hair or whatever. Having a wheelchair hasn't been a great trauma—it hasn't been a great readjustment in my life because it has been a part of my life.*

James's mother was aware of his condition when he was about eighteen months old 'simply because I did not do what the rest of the fellows in the family did'. This condition progressed for the next forty or so years of James's life, though he was still 'fairly independent until I was about fourteen or fifteen. I could shower and dress and do things for myself. I only needed help getting in and out of cars.'

Although Ian had never played competitive sport before the onset of the paralysing condition when he was nineteen, he saw himself as a 'fitness freak'. He exercised and ran regularly, not only to keep fit for his job as a seaman, an occupation that demands a high degree of physical fitness, but also to please himself.

Mark was nineteen when he had a car accident on a country road 'as a result of drinking too much alcohol and driving too fast'. Mark's family lived on the land, and his father, in particular, 'found it extremely difficult to accept my disability because he is a very physical, outdoor, sporty sort of man'. Mark's father 'put a lot of emphasis on sporting activities and physical prowess'. During school days,

> *I would be out there playing football to the best of my ability, I mean I would come off really excited about the way I had played this particular day, and I would ask, 'How did I go?'. He would say, 'Okay, but what were you dreaming about in the third quarter when you dropped the mark?'. I could never really reach his expectations.*

Clearly, then, most of the men in this study had substantial involvement in physical activities for many years prior to the onset of their disability. Many played formal competitive sport, while others spent most of their leisure time participating in vigorous physical activities of all kinds. Sports such as football, squash, badminton, tennis and cricket were enthusiastically pursued by many of the men. Others put their energies, and a great deal of their time, into more individual physical activities such as windsurfing, water-skiing and surfing. While the only man who saw himself as 'just a spectator' was severely physically restricted by his disability, most of the men professed to have been very interested in all aspects of physical activity for most of their lives. Driving cars fast, often accompanied by alcohol use, was a significant aspect of the lifestyles of many of the men, and one that directly contributed to the injuries of several of them. What then of the women in this study? Was physical activity a dominating component of the women's lives, as it was for the men?

Although Jenny

> *wasn't a sportswoman, I mean I wasn't into competitive sports or anything like that, I was active, that's why I was on the roof* [the site of her accident]. *As an adolescent I hadn't been into physical things, but the summer of my accident I had been sailing—out and about in storms or whatever. At twenty-seven I saw myself as, well, young, attractive, slim and physically . . . yeah, reasonably physically fit. I was not the sort of person who would go skydiving, but I would do something within my fears.*

Joy, too, claims that 'I am not sport oriented, I never have been even when I was younger'. However, her first job on leaving school was at a horse stud: 'I wanted to be a jockey—horses were just so important to me. I had ridden horses all my life.' The work did not last long however, and Joy 'ended up running away from home when I was about sixteen'. At the age of twenty-three, she lost control of the car she was driving on a country road. She suffered fractures to many parts of her body, including the spinal column, which injured her spinal cord in the mid-thoracic area.

Mary and her husband led

> *a pretty active life. My husband was a cyclist. It was his main sport. He raced bikes in England, though not professionally. And I'd belonged to a cycle club in England simply because I wanted to see more. We did a lot of touring in Britain and Europe before we came out here, and we did a lot of touring in the country around where we lived in Australia.*

But although Mary claims that her husband was 'a mad keen cyclist, and did a lot of hiking and mountain climbing' and because of him she became 'a sort of outdoors person', she continued to enjoy her former, more sedentary pursuits: 'I loved reading, I quite enjoyed gardening, I enjoyed walking, I enjoyed cycling, I enjoyed travelling, I enjoyed friends and I enjoyed shopping and dancing— dancing very much.' Mary and her husband were riding their tandem bicycle on a summer's evening when they were hit by an elderly motorist who had spent the afternoon in the local pub. Her husband died of head injuries within a few hours of the accident; Mary, aged thirty-four at the time and a mother of three children under the age of four, spent the next fourteen months in a rehabilitation unit.

Pam says: 'As a teenager, I was sport mad and I was music mad.' Pam was driving when she had the car accident that crushed her spinal cord. At the time, the youngest of Pam's three children was twenty months old. She had just begun to resume her interests in music and sport. Pam says: 'I had just got back to playing A-grade competitive tennis. I had also joined the Gilbert and Sullivan Society, and had gone back into one of my great areas of interest, the stage.'

Bridget was a passenger in a car that overturned on a country road, one week after she had completed her matriculation and graduated from high school. Discussing her school days Bridget says: 'I have good memories of when I played netball and softball—and of going on a speedboat and skiing and things like that.'

Sally became a paraplegic at the age of nineteen when she was a passenger in a car involved in a head-on collision with a truck. Waterskiing was her particular love: 'I started when I was four years old. Oh, I don't know if I was an expert. I've never bothered to compete. I was not really interested in competing. But I was certainly very capable. That is probably my biggest loss.' Most weekends were spent on the river, waterskiing and swimming with her three brothers and their friends. Physical activities have always been very important to Sally.

Frances is the only woman in the study who acquired her paralysis as the result of an infection, although Ian became paralysed in a similar manner. She saw herself as 'a healthy, thirty-year-old mother of three young children under five' at the time of the medical catastrophe that caused her physical losses. Frances lived with her family on a property where they were

> *into self-sufficiency—growing all our own vegetables, doing the fencing. It was a very hilly property, so I was very physically active. I had done a lot of canoeing, sailing, taking kids on expeditions. I have a very clear memory of the year I got this—I had spent the summer with the kids at a beach resort, surfing all summer. Two days before the first symptoms appeared I remember one of my friends saying, 'Go away—you look so disgustingly fit that I can't bear you to be around!'. I was very physically fit.*

Rosemary was born with the condition that caused her bodily paralysis. She attended regular secondary school, and remembers her school days, if not with happiness, then at least without rancour: 'On sports day they ran a special sixty-metre wheelchair race because there were five or six students in wheelchairs. They arranged special runs for us, but I couldn't do normal sports classes.' Rosemary has played wheelchair basketball, and has tried archery in the past. But although she does not play sport now, Rosemary is a sports enthusiast. When asked what she does in her leisure time she says: 'Football, football, football! I barrack for Carlton and the Adelaide Crows and Glenelg, of course.'

Ruth's disability was also congenital. She can remember asking her mother: ' "Why can't I run like the other kids, why can't I jump like the other kids?" ' Ruth remembers that her mother 'fobbed [her] off because she was acting on what she thought was the appropriate way of handling the situation which was don't make a big deal of it, you know, don't make an issue of it, don't treat her any differently.' Ruth has vivid memories of

> *living in fear and trepidation of sports days and of being asked to do anything physical. I was always the odd kid out. I remember when my father brought home a big skipping rope which meant that I was in control of the game. I could dictate what we played and what we did. I had some power in it, so I made sure that we did the ones [the skipping routines] that I could manage.*

Alison's condition meant that she spent the early part of her life in an institution. Although she has used an electric wheelchair for the last fifteen years, she managed a regular wheelchair before that time. She claims that her 'physical capabilities are, in fact, much better now that I am out in the normal community because the range of things I have to do is much more expanded than if I were sitting in an institution'. Tina received the diagnosis of her progressive condition at the age of three, some thirty years ago. By the age of eighteen the condition had deteriorated to the extent that she required a wheelchair all of the time. Robyn, in her late fifties, is the oldest person in this study. Robyn's lateness in achieving the usual milestones of childhood development led to a firm diagnosis of her condition at about eighteen months of age. She was unable to walk unaided until the age of five, and by the age of seven needed calipers and sticks in order to walk with any degree of functional success. Robyn says: 'Balance was a problem. I was always excused from marching and things like that, but I was usually included in games with other kids.' She has been in a wheelchair for the last eight or nine years.

These data suggest two main conclusions. First, although the women's previous involvement in physical activities was nowhere near as formal or long-standing as that of the men in this study, many of the women were in fact quite physically active and prided themselves on 'being fit'. Although several of the women played sports such as tennis, netball and softball, many of them had strong commitments to less organised, more individualised activities such as cycling, sailing, dancing, walking, waterskiing, surfing and canoeing. Rosemary, who has been paralysed since birth, pushes her wheelchair around the block several times each day for exercise, and her consuming passion in life is that of a football spectator. The importance of *general physical capabilities* was often expressed by even the most severely paralysed women.

Second, the women did not pursue the activities with the same sense of 'naturalness' that was assumed by the men, nor did the women's activities appear to be as substantially developed or to have the same long-established nature as those pursued by the men. Certainly many men cease to participate in formal sport at an early age, but their interest in things physical seems abiding. Some of the women had developed their interest in their physical activity at a relatively late stage in life, or in response to their partner's or family's interests. When undertaken by women, the physical activities seemed to have a 'temporary tenure'. In contrast, the physical activities discussed by the men seemed to be integrated into their whole lives. Sport related with other aspects of their lives—their work, their leisure, their 'lifestyle', their sense of self—in a seamless manner. Changing from one sport to another, from competitive sport to more individualistic physical activity, from participator to spectator status, from doer to talker—was simply a new aspect of the fundamental physicality of the body. The primacy of physicality in the social construction of masculinity was not threatened by such superficial changes in expression.

Some of the women were very committed to sport, but their activities appeared to have a different relationship to their lives. The women often became involved with an activity because of a partner's prior interest in that activity. Jenny, for example, began sailing because of a partner's involvement. Mary became skilled in bicycling because of her husband's excellence in competitive cycling. Frances's enjoyment of water sports and her commitment to the hard work of self-sufficiency farming fitted into the needs of her marriage and family life. Sally's waterskiing was compatible with the interests of her family. This complementary nature of women's interest in sporting and physical activities seems quite different from men's relationship with their physical activities. The women's physical activities relate to other people's interests, rather than being 'pure interests' of their own. This 'fitting in with others', the complementary nature of women's participation, is quite different from the 'stand alone' character of men's participation (Deem 1987, pp. 210–28; Griffin et al. 1982, pp. 88–117). Men may invite women to join them in their activities, but they would do them anyway, often with other men.

Not only are the women's activities characterised by a quality of 'fitting in', but the women often describe such activities as 'keeping fit'. Women's engagement in sport is likely to be more pragmatically motivated. Women exercise to 'be fit', 'to keep in shape'. Women are much less likely to be enmeshed in physicality than men; their relationship is more practical. Women's physical activities may be related to health concerns—to received wisdoms associated with the connection between exercise and health status (Lenskyj 1986, ch. 1; Matthews 1987, p. 18). Alternatively, or as well, women may engage in physical activity in order 'to look good' (Matthews 1987, p. 18)—a motivation directed at others, though doubtless a woman will also please herself by pleasing others. As Mary says: 'I appreciated very much losing a lot of weight when I became more active, and being able to wear nice clothes that looked good. I was very conscious of what I bought. I still am.'

Not least, a woman may engage in physical activity in order to enhance or maintain her capacity to physically care for others: 'If I don't keep fit then who will look after them?' In contrast with men's enduring relationship with physical activities throughout their lives, women's connection is more temporary. Women's interests seem to move from one activity to another. Each new interest seems to be a separate issue in their lives, unlike the case of men, for whom it constitutes another new element in the seamless flow of physicality. Women's relationship with physicality is different. Though very important for the women, sport and physical activities remained a 'thing apart'—separable from their lives, yet closely tied to the lives of others.

THE REHABILITATION PROGRAM

What of the rehabilitation program itself? Sport and the ideology of athleticism are critical components of the formal rehabilitation project. Most of the informants, those men and women whose paralyses result from spinal injuries, have spent a considerable time as residents in a spinal injuries rehabilitation unit. The remaining informants have spent many years of their lives attending rehabilitation programs on a regular basis, or living in an institution. As the name implies, rehabilitation is concerned with the restoration of the injured person into society. Less acknowledged, but much more important, is the reconstitution of self-identity in relation to the person's new bodily state—the process of re-embodiment. This process may take a very long time and, indeed, may never occur, but critical elements of this project derive from the informants' early experiences in a formal rehabilitation context.

The Stoke Mandeville Spinal Injuries Centre in England was opened in 1944 in anticipation of war casualties with injuries to the spinal cord. These casualties were, almost exclusively, men. The program initiated at Stoke Mandeville has been the model for spinal injuries centres throughout the world. Sir Ludwig Guttman, the Foundation Director of the Stoke Mandeville Centre, was a persuasive proponent of such rehabilitation. His prolific writings on the subject in academic publications, and his consultative visits with regard to the creation and management of spinal units, propagated the influence of the Stoke Mandeville model of spinal injuries rehabilitation throughout the world (Seymour 1989, p. 56). Guttman's influence was not diminished by his death in 1980. With minor variations, units closely resembling the basic concept of Stoke Mandeville exist in many parts of the world, and in most States of Australia (Guttman 1967, pp. 115–26; 1973, ch. 3).

It is not hard to identify the associations with masculinity embedded in the foundations of spinal injuries rehabilitation. War is the primary arena of physical challenge. Aggression and defence, gains and losses, tactical moves, strategic plans, bravery, heroism, resistance, attack, victory, capitulation and defeat are the activities and the vernacular of war. With little modification, the metaphors and activities of real warfare become transposed to mock battles on the sports arena (Elias & Dunning 1986). Battlefields for the defence of suburban values replaced the fields of war. Deeply embedded values, attitudes and expressions are reinforced in the 'play fights', as they were in the deadly serious conflicts between nations. Displays of physical strength and feats of endurance valorised in warfare are similarly rewarded on the sports field. Just as the 'character building' and the disciplinary aspects of war service were valued, sport too is seen to inculcate these critical characteristics in its adherents. Spectators and supporters on the side lines are vital not only to the success of each game, but also to the continual reaffirmation of the key values of masculinity upon which sport is based. War, sport, physicality and masculinity share particular attributes and values. Playing sport, like going to war, will 'make a boy a man'. Sporting heroes, like war heroes, embody much that is valued in society.

Not surprisingly, then, these values formed the foundation of spinal injury rehabilitation at Stoke Mandeville. Men injured in the selfless defence of their country deserved the best rehabilitation that the country could provide. The key values of war were transformed into the dominant themes of bodily rehabilitation. Men's bodily damage sustained in physical combat while engaged in national defence, a political cause traditionally seen as men's business, demanded similarly masculinist treatment. Sport provided an opportunity for them to continue to reaffirm the key values of masculinity. Injuries caused by the physicality of war were, in peacetime, managed by the physicality of rehabilitation.

Thus, sport has been an essential component of rehabilitation since the inception of the Stoke Mandeville Centre. The social and psychological advantages of participation in sport were considered equal to its immense physical benefits for people with physical disability (Seymour 1989, p. 56). The first Stoke Mandeville Games took place in 1948. In 1952 these games became an international event and they are now held annually either at Stoke Mandeville or in the country hosting the Olympic Games (Guttman 1967, p. 125).

Battle analogies are often heard in a rehabilitation setting, as they are in discourses related to cancer and AIDS (Lupton 1994, p. 61). Injunctions to 'fight the disease', 'conquer the disability', 'battle against the losses' and 'overcome the odds' reflect an approach to a war that must be fought, not against an alien oppressor, but against the person's own body. Formal rehabilitation work is work on the body. It is only by intensive concentration of energy and unremitting work on the body over a very long time that the paralysed person will be able to manage those activities of the body that have been cut adrift from their central control. Successful body work is the key to liberation (Seymour 1989, p. 60).

Such single-minded devotion to the physical body clearly fits better within masculinity than within the social category of femininity. Men's life-long association with physical activities and sport places them at a distinct advantage in terms of the outcomes of rehabilitation. Not only are men more inclined to respond to the physical nature of rehabilitation, but also, when rehabilitated, their bodies will present an image to the world that fits a powerful physical definition of masculinity. Such definition may override other aspects of the man's body where his masculinity has been threatened. Work, sexuality and fathering a child, for example, may be severely challenged by the injury, but activities that build the muscles of the upper trunk, shoulders and arms may well serve to mask these losses, at least in the eyes of others (Seymour 1989, p. 114).

Although a well-developed upper body would clearly also have important functional advantages for women with paraplegia, a visible presentation of physical strength and power is antithetical to femininity. While success in sport is success in being masculine, the situation is quite the opposite for women (Willis 1982, p. 123; Hargreaves 1986, p. 153). The woman may lose more than she gains from such a body, and the unremitting physical work that she would have to pursue to build her body in this way would divert her energies from other activities where her self-identity would be better served. Although some women athletes are beginning to challenge the rigid dimensions of 'ideal' body shape, the struggles of women like body-builder Bev Francis reinforce the immense difficulties involved in attempting to change the boundaries of strength and acceptable appearance for women (Bryson 1987, p. 356; Steinem 1994, pp. 93–122).

Clearly the opportunities for physical activities are much better for people with paraplegia than for people with quadriplegia. Although a quadriplegic, Anthony claims that he 'spent a lot of hours doing physical stuff—I was oriented towards it, it was familiar ground to me. I found it to be a good escape out of the unit. You could push yourself harder into physiotherapy, hydro and gym stuff.' However Anthony says that he 'found it very frustrating. It was very difficult to get satisfaction out of it compared to my framework of what was satisfying before.'

Anthony's sense of being 'second class' in terms of his previous physical competence was compounded by what he describes as the elitism of the gym staff favouring people who have suffered less physical loss: 'Games can be adapted more easily for people who have more physical abilities, and they can be more competitive.' The paradox of this is clear. Energy and attention are directed to those paralysed people who, while needing it, need it less than those people with far greater physical loss. Anthony says that attempts to redress this rehabilitative paradox have been occurring over the last four or five years as games that are satisfying and competitive for people with severe spinal injuries, 'not just the functionally elite', are being explored and developed.

Bob, a paraplegic, was one of the 'functionally elite' in Anthony's terms. Sport had been an important part of his past, and was to play a large part in his rehabilitation. Bob claims that he 'got encouraged a lot in sport' while he was in the unit: 'I remember going to the gymnasium and practising basketball. I missed the ring by about four feet. I'd fall backward in the chair if I threw too hard. The healthier I got the more mobile I got and the more bored I got. I did my routine rehab stuff, but I wanted to do more—so I used to go to the gym a lot to practise.' Bob's interest in sport was also an important source of sociability. Groups would form around this shared interest. 'We would all get in one room with our chairs up against the door so noone could come in. We'd have fun—talk, a few drinks, a lot of sharing of knowledge, asking questions.'

The practical reality of having to lift your body around on your arms after these paralysing injuries means that prior involvement in sport, or being 'sports minded' will greatly facilitate the rehabilitation process. Although Bob now claims that 'there has to be room for people who are not sports minded—being physically active is not the only way out of here', he is quite unequivocal in attributing his rehabilitative success to sport and its role in providing his pathway out of the rehabilitation unit. The fact that 'they emphasised sport and I was a bit of a sportsman before, meant that I left the unit in September and went to the National Games in Perth in November of the same year. I played B-grade basketball. I had a go at every race in track, and I came last in every race.'

Mark spent eighteen months in the spinal injuries unit. Although his experience was more than twenty years ago, he too remembers the dominating influence of physicality during this time:

> There was a lot of emphasis on sporting activities and strong encouragement to become part of the paraplegic sport events and to get into sporting activities. A lot of emphasis was put on weight-lifting in both physiotherapy and in sports therapy. I got right into all of that. A bit of sprinting, javelin, the shot-put, swimming, basketball—yes, that was the most exciting one, I used to enjoy that the most.

Mark talks of the conflicting tensions associated with his participation in sport at this time:

I wanted to be involved with other people with disabilities, to develop an identity and a sense of belonging, but at the same time I did not want to be part of that—I wanted to be separate from them. I did not have much in common with a lot of the people involved. What we had in common was the fact that we had the same disability.

As a quadriplegic, there was no sport that Peter could play during his time in the rehabilitation unit seven or eight years ago.

Sport is offered through the gym instructors. Depending on whether a person is a paraplegic or a quadriplegic determines how far they can go in wheelchair sports. If a person is in an electric wheelchair he doesn't have a high hope—there are not many sports that he can participate in. Blow darts is an option, but that is about all.

Blow darts was not an option that appealed to Peter at the time, but he, too, considered that ideas and values about playing sport were strongly articulated in the routine gym work at the unit, and that this way of thinking was very influential in later ideas about playing sport as both exercise and leisure.

The masculine character of the rehabilitation unit seems well established by these reports. Gymnasium work, weight-lifting, physiotherapy, transfers and the learning of wheelchair skills take place in a residential context in which the patients are overwhelmingly young and male, and the staff are overwhelmingly young and female (Seymour 1989, p. 62). The emphasis on body building and on sport, and on particular kinds of sport, is masculine in orientation. When discussing the ways his fellow rehabilitatees used their bodies in the rehabilitation unit, Ken says 'some of these younger guys think that they are invulnerable'—an ironic remark in light of the reality of their extensive bodily damage, yet strong confirmation of the enduring power of masculine ideas about the body. The preferencing of the physical body in men's lives prepares them for the physical nature of rehabilitation and the physicality of the rehabilitation unit. Men who are less involved in the world of sport will find the process more difficult. Women may be disadvantaged by the physical nature of rehabilitation.

When asked to comment on how they thought women with spinal injuries would fare in the rehabilitation context, many of the male informants told me about a particular woman with paraplegia 'who was very involved in gym work, who developed a lot of skills and who ended up being a very good basketballer'. So often was this woman cited that it became clear to me that her achievements had attained legendary status in rehabilitation lore. Clearly her physical achievements were exceptional in terms of women's rehabilitation.

By chance, I found myself conducting an interview with an informant who was clearly the exceptional sportswoman whom I had heard mentioned so often in my interviews with the men. Sally was very involved in sport before her accident. Her love of water-skiing has been documented earlier in this chapter. At the time of her accident, Sally had just finished the second year of her registered nursing training, ironically as a staff member of the spinal injuries unit. Nevertheless Sally describes the unit as a 'terrible place, it's something out of history, it felt like you were back in World War II. I just wanted to get out of there as quickly as I could. Fortunately I knew how to do that with the knowledge that I have of spinal injuries.'

When asked to explain her statement that the unit was a masculine environment, Sally said:

> Guys really don't mind what's around them as much as a woman. Part of a woman being a woman is where she is and what is around her and her control of that—and there was none of that. Chauvinism is possibly a little bit unfair, but I think the guys get better treatment. The fact that more guys go through than women means that it is more oriented towards men, and therefore the chauvinism actually thrives. The staff are fine, but they are mainly women, and they love attending men.

Although interactions were usually gendered in the manner described above, Sally goes on to say:

> I used to get a lot of attention when I went to weights or to the gym area because there were two guys working there. They loved working with women, I mean that is a novelty to them. You get a lot of attention and they look after you, but they never pushed me or made the demands from me that they would have made from a guy in the same situation.

Despite her success, Sally was indignant about what she saw as the differential treatment of men and women: 'They try hard and expect more from a guy than a woman, which is wrong. Their attitude is that this is a bit of fun for you, but deadly earnest for a guy. Why shouldn't I be able to do everything that a guy can do in the same situation when I got out of that place? I needed to.'

Though her experience of a spinal injury unit occurred a few years later, Jenny's memories of the rehabilitation context have many similarities with Sally's: 'I have memories of things like the weight-lifting men who were very masculine, physical, phys. ed. sort of guys. The way they pranced around was pretty sexist.' Jenny goes on to say:

> There is another division in there that they actually promote, and I was on the positive side of it because I was a paraplegic. There were only two paraplegics in the unit whereas there were seventeen quadriplegics. I was able to do the physical weight-lifting and strenuous activities which was what made you acceptable to them. So that became not so much a gender issue as a physical capacity issue. And in some ways I actually developed a sense of satisfaction about being able to weight-lift for the first time, and discover some new parts of me around that.

Although Jenny's claim that these issues were influenced more by physical capacity than gender has some validity, gender clearly underlies the values associated with physical performance in this context, and also the sense of delight that Jenny experienced in discovering aspects of her body that are denied women in more usual contexts. But although Jenny remembers the powerful presence of the male gym instructors during her time in the unit, she claims that the system is controlled by the male orderlies: 'Their subculture dominates significantly, and I don't think that this should be underestimated.'

As discussed before, a spinal injuries unit provides services to many more men than women because men engage in the kind of physical activities that endanger their spinal cord, and clearly, rehabilitation is also dominated by masculine ideas and values. The built environment is masculine, the culture is masculine, rehabilitation plans are presented in terms of gender assumptions about men and women, progress and success are judged in masculine terms, and rehabilitation projections reflect fixed and static views of men's and women's roles. Not surprisingly women, and of course some men, feel uncomfortable in this context.

While defending the rehabilitation unit against gender bias, Peter demonstrated some of the very contradictions and opacities that support the reality he is attempting to deny. Peter claims that 'it is important for your self-esteem to play sport because it is seen as an important way of showing masculinity. I feel that if women are able to, then they are equally steered along that path and support is given for them to do some sport because it is very helpful.' Even though he agrees that body building might not fit conventional notions of femininity, Peter feels 'that in a wheelchair different rules apply. A woman is seen as being an athlete in a wheelchair, irrespective of whether she is a male or a female. It is seen as opposite to femininity, but I don't feel that people go looking at that. They see the wheelchair first, not her muscles.'

Peter's explanation denies the different relationship of men and women to their physical bodies and the implications of this in terms of the past experiences, orientations, associated values and abilities that they bring to the task of re-embodiment. Men and women do not begin rehabilitation on neutral terms. Men are enormously advantaged in terms of the physical nature of masculinity; even those men who 'have never played sport in their lives' benefit from this association. In addition to this opacity, however, is an even more damaging deduction. For a woman, sport and a wheelchair are associations that appear to eradicate gender all together. The social category of athlete and the social ideas associated with a wheelchair transcend womanliness. The woman is effectively eliminated. Femaleness disappears in the face of the dominance of the masculinity–physicality connection. There is no doubt, however, that masculinity is strongly reinforced by sport.

Such differences are critical issues in rehabilitation as it is presently constituted. Weight-lifting and training are clearly of immense practical importance in preparing the undamaged parts of the body to do the work of those parts of the body that have been lost. If paralysed people can maintain their physical strength and abilities through regular participation in sport, the boredom of solitary gymnasium work can be minimised in favour of competitive, goal-directed activities in which interaction with others, bonding, confidence, assertiveness, discipline and endurance will emerge. Interest in paraplegic sport, like interest in regular sport, guarantees entry into male culture with all its attendant benefits.

INVOLVEMENT IN SPORT BEYOND THE UNIT

Disparities of power between the client and the worker in the enclosed world of the rehabilitation unit, the physical vulnerabilities of the newly disabled person, and the catastrophic nature of the situation may well contribute to initial compliance with this physical model of rehabilitation. But what happens when people leave the rehabilitation context? Does the strong focus on physicality survive beyond the unit, and do male advantages continue?

Physical activity is now David's full-time career. A sports club devoted to people with body paralyses, which he joined some twenty years ago, has occupied much of his time. Not only did it provide him with the opportunity to compete with others in sporting contests, but the club was also an important source of social contacts. Compensation from the accident released him from the need to work for several years and enabled David to become even more involved with the sports club. It was this close association that led to the job of which he now speaks with such enthusiasm. He says:

> I thoroughly enjoy this job. It is an extremely satisfying position because I work with people that I can probably understand more than most of the other staff. You do get depressing moments when you get some bad quadriplegics through. We have close links with the sports association which I am still heavily involved with. I am a life member and vice president. I can do my training here. I get time off to go overseas. Since I have been involved with the sports association I have been overseas fourteen times.

David is a world-standard wheelchair basketballer. Yet he says that it took him a long time before he developed the attitude compatible with playing wheelchair sport:

> It's just as competitive as any other sport, but you have to deal with the ignorance of people who are not aware of that. People pat you on the back and say, 'Good on you boys', and 'Good to see you out of hospital today!'. Even after working here for more than ten years I still get asked, 'What room are you in?' or 'Did they bring you in an ambulance?'.

Success in disabled sport, unlike success in able-bodied sport, is not associated with mastery in other dimensions of life. Achievement in wheelchair sport does not have the power to transform the primary status, that of patient. Disabled sport remains sport for people with damaged bodies. The treatment of the Paralympics by people associated with the regular Olympics is instructive in this regard. It may be 'just as competitive as any other sport', as David claims, but the competition is seen as particular, and the social rewards remain circumscribed within this particularity. George confirms this when he says that although he 'shoots', and is 'trying to organise a new sport for quads called wheelchair rugby', he tries to keep friendships developed through these associations 'to a minimum, otherwise you get stuck in a rut. I want to avoid that. You don't want to close yourself off, to be stuck for the rest of your life.'

Peter, like George, is a quadriplegic, and he too is involved in wheelchair rugby. This sport, which originated in Canada and was introduced to Australia around 1990, is played using similar rules to wheelchair basketball, except that scoring involves moving through the goals in the chair rather than shooting baskets. Peter says:

Unfortunately it is a very elitist sport, even for quadriplegics, because there are only a very small number of quadriplegics with lesions low enough to be able to take up the game. If the lesion is any higher they would not have the manoeuvrability or the ability to actually do the movements needed to pick up the ball and things like that.

What satisfactions could this game bring to a man who had spent most of his life on the back of a horse? Peter describes the prestige associated with wheelchair sport: 'Wheelchair sport has such a high reputation. I feel good about being part of wheelchair sport because it is an elitist place to be—rather than just being a person in a wheelchair. Playing sport is very good for your attitude and your self-esteem.'

The gender and functional biases inherent in the wheelchair sports association were Gerald's particular frustration. He says, 'It concentrates on young active males, and doesn't concern itself with people in wheelchairs with other disabilities, or with women.' Gerald, too, refers to Sally's exceptional sporting talents:

Sally was the only woman who participated to any extent. She became 'one of the boys'—she played basketball as hard as they did, she was much better than most of them. She got into the State team, and that caused a lot of friction. Was it really a men's basketball competition or was it a wheelchair sport competition? Should she be allowed to compete?

Although Ken was a very committed surfer before his accident he claims that he has 'never been interested in gym and weights and that kind of thing. I did it through my rehabilitation because I had to get my strength back on.' Ken now plays wheelchair basketball on two nights of the week. When asked at what level he played the game Ken replied:

I guess I don't have any ambition to play for the State or for Australia because I am never going to be that good. I am not prepared to put in the amount of work that is necessary to be that good. I look at people like [names three men who have achieved excellence in wheelchair sport]—I mean they spend half of their lives training. They get out there and they do the hard work, and good luck to them, but I have no aspirations in that direction. I play wheelchair basketball more as a leisure activity than anything, and as an attempt to keep my weight down, although I don't think that it is very successful.

During his time in the rehabilitation unit, Mark pursued physical activities with great enthusiasm: 'There was a lot of emphasis on sporting activities. We used to play table tennis for hours on end, so much so that I developed an aversion to the sound of table tennis balls bouncing on the table.' Mark says that although he 'got right into paraplegic sporting activities then', he doesn't have any involvement with sporting activities now. He says:

> I used to feel that I had some obligation to be involved, so I used to go and play basketball and those things even though I didn't necessarily enjoy a lot of the politics on the way—the interactions that occurred. I didn't have a lot in common with a lot of the people involved. What we had in common was the fact that we had the same disability. Towards the end of my involvement with the sporting club I remember having this sense of 'What am I doing this for?'—What am I getting out of it?'.

Despite this latter-day evaluation however, Mark involved himself in paraplegic sport for nearly ten years. He is clear in acknowledging his enjoyment of the competition involved in this activity and the opportunity it gave him to keep fit.

Before his diving accident at the age of nineteen, sporting activities took up most of Ron's non-working life. This active involvement has now been converted into a spectator's interest. Ron says 'I watch as much sport as I can. I go to sporting events if I can, weather permitting. If it is a nice day I'll go.'

The evidence indicates that the physical model of rehabilitation serves men well initially, though of course it is more beneficial for men with lower [paraplegic] than higher [quadriplegic] lesions. Not only is the strong focus on physicality harder to sustain beyond this point, but retaining this orientation may well impede re-embodiment for men, as well as for women, despite its obvious functional advantages.

Mary has never played wheelchair sport. She likes swimming, but finds that it is a bit of a hassle to find somewhere to go. Mary explains: 'With my pressure problems [skin breakdown] I am not prepared to drag myself over the side of a swimming pool. And where is there a place nearby with a hoist?' Maintaining the strength of the upper body is a constant concern for paralysed people. Mary says, 'I push up and down Northridge Road, which is very steep. I need to do this regularly to develop my shoulders.' Rosemary has tried some wheelchair sport, but is not really interested in active involvement with these activities. Like Ron, her involvement in sport is that of a spectator: she is a passionate football supporter, rarely missing a match. In summer, though, she enjoys 'going to the beach with my friends. We try to stay on the wet, hard sand because the wheelchair becomes bogged so easily in the soft sand.' Although Rosemary can't swim, she enjoys the water by kneeling in it. She too, like Mary, 'walks' around the block twice a day to maintain the strength of her back, shoulders and arms.

Sally's relationship with sport is legendary: even within this chapter her sporting achievements and her attitudes towards physicality have taken a leading role. Compensation from the accident together with wise investments have meant that Sally has been able to work on a very part-time basis and have the time 'to play sport, to swim, canoe, sailboard and camp and all those type of things which I enjoy'. Sally continues:

> *At the moment I am really involved with basketball. I train with the guys' team. We play like the 36ers play their home and away games, once a week, and we train with them twice a week. I play every Sunday night in the local competition, two games on each Sunday night—and this is basically off season, so it is quiet at the moment. When I am training up to a tournament or a game, I tend to train eight or nine sessions a week.*

Sally acknowledges that she plays more sport than any other woman in a wheelchair. She says that there are a few men who play as much or more sport than she does: 'I am the only woman who is competing at the same level as the guys. I have been doing this for about eight to ten years—and for that length of time I have been trying to develop women's basketball. There was no women's basketball until about three years ago, and finally I got it off the ground.' Before this Sally played 'with the guys, which meant that I could only compete to Australian level, I could not compete for Australia internationally'. Now Sally has the additional advantage of international travel, as well as the benefits she gains from the physical exercise and the competition. She considers that sport has been the key factor in her re-embodiment: 'You get the best feed-back on doing the right thing—all the positives.' Sally is well aware that 'for most women, sport takes on a very minor, leisure time role in their lives, whereas in my life, since the accident, it has been central. If I were an able-bodied woman I may not have had the opportunity.' Sally is also clear that her financial security and her involvement in sport have enabled her to avoid the issue of work: a difficulty for all people with disabilities, but especially for women. The women with children, or those in less stable financial circumstances, were unable to utilise this pathway of re-embodiment.

ADVANTAGES AND DISADVANTAGES OF
THE PHYSICAL MODEL

The enormous obstacles many men have had to overcome to become wheelchair athletes must not be underestimated. The excellence achieved by competitors in the Paralympic Games and other similar contests is a resounding testimony to human ability and determination in the face of extreme adversity. Australia's success in the ninth Paralympic Games in Barcelona in 1992 renewed enthusiasm for the event; the marathon was described by many spectators and sportswriters as a 'more remarkable event than the '92 Olympics' (Griffiths 1992, p. 25). The Atlanta Paralympics in 1996 compounded the success of the previous games. A winning wheelchair athlete is seen as the epitome of rehabilitative success. The vision of strong male bodies competing for honours on the sports field is an image that has currency in the able-bodied world. Bravery in overcoming the catastrophe of a damaged body is a quality everyone can admire.

While the benefits to these people may be immense, many other people with severe, permanent disability are damaged by the predominance of this model of rehabilitation. I have already cited Anthony's views of what he calls the 'elitism' of the gym staff who manage this important part of the rehabilitation process. Because of the high prestige of physicality in the construction of masculinity, and the critical role of sport as the vehicle of masculine physicality, the energy of the rehabilitative task is directed at those people with less physical loss: a 'functional elite'. Attention is directed at those people who have suffered the least loss. Professional rewards are enhanced by this process, but such strategies are also motivated by altruism. In order to create areas of success for those people who have lost so much, it is not surprising that staff may single out those people who have most potential for development. The creation of role models may be even more important in this context than in the everyday world where a broader range of choices are available; although ironically, recent research has indicated that the 'trickledown' effect of sporting excellence by top-level athletes may hinder, rather than foster, attempts to promote participation at the grassroots level (Hindson & Gidlow 1994, p. 11).

Clearly, paraplegic men are the beneficiaries of this rehabilitative focus. But many paraplegic men may not value sport so highly, nor be prepared to engage in the single-minded and unremitting work needed to train the body for participation in competition at this level. While the men may be immersed in the world of sport as observers, they may simply not be interested in active physical exercise for themselves. Thinking about sport, in this context as in the able-bodied world, may be more important for many men than playing it. While a familiarity with physicality and its associated ideas and attitudes will advantage men in rehabilitation, this familiarity, on its own, will not build strong muscles.

Men with quadriplegia—paralysis of all four limbs and a large part of the trunk—are unlikely to benefit directly from this rehabilitative focus. While their physical losses are far more extensive than those of people with paraplegia, and thus their need for thoroughgoing and creative rehabilitative options is far greater, these people may be viewed as having 'little potential' because they cannot participate in the physical orientation of a rehabilitation unit. The preferencing of physicality in spinal injuries rehabilitation may disenfranchise the very people who most need its services. The creation of sporting heroes as rehabilitative triumphs obliterates from view the many severely damaged people for whom such activities will always be an impossibility.

Even men who have never played sport or who profess disinterest in physical activities will benefit from the ideas about men's bodies that have informed their perceptions about themselves and the way they are seen by others from childhood. Of course, countless examples exist of able-bodied women who have achieved excellence in physical arenas. In this study related to damaged bodies, Sally clearly is an example of excellence. Yet in the face of the dominant construction of femininity, women's bodies simply cannot embody the qualities necessary to achieve success in these activities. Success is seen as exceptional, rather than generally possible.

The advantages of strongly developed upper-body muscles for people with bodily paralyses have been discussed before. Yet the cost of such freedom may outweigh the losses in relation to the dominant constructions of femininity. Well-developed shoulders, neck and back may also lift the woman out of the category 'female' and place her in the social category 'athlete'. 'Athlete', as we have explored, is a masculine term. Physicality and femininity are antithetical. The unquestionable advantages of physical development and sporting activities for people with damaged bodies may be simply too costly for women.

Mary bemoans what she claims 'are my huge shoulders. They were big anyway, but with all this physical stuff they have become enormous. I am not as well developed as some wheelchair users. I have had to go into T shirts and these lovely batwing jumpers and things. I've got some nice blouses down there that I can't wear any more.' Mary is fully aware of the necessity 'to live with my shoulders now', but has many regrets about the changes that strenthening her upper body has made to her appearance.

Pam, too, grieves at the changes that physical rehabilitation has wrought on her body:

Suddenly you haven't got that nice shape and that waistline. Your shoulders and arms are hyper-developed because they have to take the whole workload of the body. When I was going through the continual physiotherapy and weight-lifting programs they used to tell women that if they wanted to develop their bustlines that this was the way to go.

Even in a situation where physical development can make the difference between independence or dependence on others, women still have to be coaxed into such activities with the sugar-coated pill of breast enhancement. Breast development serves no purpose but to please others. Body development enables the woman to help herself.

When discussing the issue of breast development, Sally says: 'I mean to some degree it can be feminine, but the muscle bulk goes on in such a way that is not quite feminine because it's all in your shoulders and around your bust. I'm big enough there as it is, so that detracts from my appearance.' Sally considers that this type of body building 'is not attractive at all. It emphasises the fact that you are big and bulky at the top, and the fact that I carry extra weight makes it ten times worse, not just twice as bad.'

Despite such damning comments, however, when asked if she had ever considered these issues to be sufficient grounds for exercising less, Sally replied:

No, exercise is too important—vitally, absolutely important. I think that it is important for able-bodied people too, but just that much more for someone in a chair. It is not just physically important for me, but mentally. Anyone in a chair who does not play some sort of sport or do something physical starts to look like a crip, rather than looking like someone who is disabled.

Sally goes on to talk about a woman she had met the night before whom 'I used to play sport with and who used to look so healthy and vital. Even though she married and had two kids she still used to look really healthy and vital. But now she has stopped playing sport, and she is starting to look like a woman in a chair.' Sally says that she keeps her hair long and pays attention to her fingernails in order to counteract her broad-shouldered, masculine appearance. 'Actually the thing people notice about me now is my hair. I am described as that girl in the chair with the long hair. I am lucky it's nice. It takes attention from my big shoulders, my masculine, tomboyish ways, my roughness on the basketball court.' Even though Sally gets someone to braid her hair for her when she plays basketball 'it still looks slightly feminine, and it's right off my face. I've got to prove something when I am out there, but I do pay a lot of attention to my hair and my nails because I need them to look feminine.'

Proving something on the sports field evokes the masculine, which must be countered by the assertion of feminine (Bryson 1987, p. 356; Graydon 1983, p. 8; Hargreaves 1986, p. 152; Loudon 1992, p. 21). Men's particular external bodily features are obscured by active, successful, physical activities. Certainly followers of male sporting heroes would be aware of the physical dimensions of the men, but adulation of men's features builds onto the physical success, it does not act against it. Having built up her body and achieved considerable sporting success, Sally now feels that 'I must groom myself to be more feminine. If I can be more feminine in that way then it will cover up other areas where I lack. It will also cover the fact that when I'm on the court I am so rough.' When playing sport, Sally says that she is very aggressive and very rough and certainly not at all feminine. And I don't feel feminine on the court. If you do feel it [feminine] on the court, well then you're not going to be a good basketballer.' Masculinity, it seems, is critical to physical success; femininity is its antithesis. Womanliness is subsumed by sporting success. Certainly the social category of 'wheelchair athlete' is firmly structured in terms of male paraplegia. 'The woman' effectively disappears in relation to the dominance of both 'the wheelchair' and 'the athlete'. The feminine is neutralised by the established power of the masculinity–physicality nexus. A woman must take extraordinary measures to direct attention to her 'feminine' attributes in order to prove to others that she can be both successful and a woman.

Sally's statement that 'anyone in a chair who does not play some sort of sport or do something physical starts to look like a crip, rather than looking like someone who is disabled' would seem to have serious implications for people who either choose against, or are unable to engage in, physical activities. Sally made a similar distinction between a woman who looked 'healthy and vital' when she played sport and on ceasing to play sport looks 'like a woman in a chair'. The distinction between 'a crip' and 'someone who is disabled' appears to be profound, as does the dichotomy between healthy vitality and being a woman in a chair. What do these distinctions imply about gender and physicality?

A crip, an abbreviation of cripple, is presumably someone with a disability who does not play sport or engage in physical activities. A person who plays sport enjoys the privileged category of a person with a disability. The ability to engage in physical activity is an important vehicle of status mobility in relation to bodily loss. One may be dismissed as a crip or may be incorporated as someone who is disabled on this basis. Of course the extent of the physical loss plays a part in this distinction, but more importantly, such discrimination arises from the physical focus of the rehabilitation project and the pre-eminence of physical achievement in this model. Similarly, health and vitality are seen to be the result of sporting activity. Health and vitality are, presumably, also linked to gender, since on ceasing to play sport the healthy, vital person with a disability begins to look like a 'woman in a chair'. The pejorative implications of this status passage are clear. Sport and physical activities enable a woman with a disability to transcend gender. Femaleness disappears in the face of the masculinity–physicality connection. On ceasing to play sport, however, a woman loses the privileged status she has enjoyed while basking in this reflected light and reverts to being merely a 'woman in a chair'.

It is easy to understand how this route may appeal to women whose remaining physical abilities enable them to pursue the option. The short-term advantages of this vicarious association may seem to offer a substantial rehabilitative pathway for some women, as it does for many men. But what must women lose in order to gain this deputed status? Must a woman lose her womanhood in order to enjoy this short-lived advantage? In accepting the path offering rehabilitative expediency, more may be lost than can be gained. Women with permanent disability have lost so much of their bodily capacity: must they also lose their gender?

It seems that few people with disabilities benefit from this model of rehabilitation. Neither the men nor the women with the extensive bodily losses associated with quadriplegia will be served by the physical focus of this model. Amongst the informants in this study, this would include Alister, Anthony, George, Peter and Ron. Most of the men and women with conditions that cause less-predictable musculoskeletal loss than do spinal injuries will be unable to engage in the type of physical activities promoted by this model. This would include Ian, James, Alison, Frances, Robyn, Ruth and Tina.

People whose bodily damage is limited to one half of the body, either upper or lower body, are clearly the beneficiaries of this form of rehabilitation. Damage to the upper body leaves the lower limbs intact to be trained for physical acts such as running, jumping or riding. Lower body loss, as in paraplegia, involves the substitution of a wheelchair for these acts of locomotion, freeing the upper body for substantial redevelopment. Seven women—Jenny, Joy, Mary, Pam, Bridget, Rosemary and Sally—and five men—Bob, Ken, David, Gerald and Mark—fit this category of bodily loss in this study. Yet, as discussed previously, the women may well lose more than they gain from physical rehabilitation. In this small study alone, then, there appear to be only five of the twenty-four informants who will benefit from this kind of rehabilitative model; yet all will be subject to its influence, and all will be evaluated in terms of its principles. Of course, privileging physicality in rehabilitative contexts merely reflects the values of the able-bodied world. No matter how well-meaning such 'normalising' may seem, however, encouragement of people with damaged bodies to aspire to the dominant values of masculine physicality must be critically examined. Enormous energy and discipline are required to create the body needed for elite wheelchair activities. The body must be retrained through countless hours of muscle building and kinesiological activity. A man's body developed in this way may present a strong image of physical masculinity, an image that may serve to deflect attention from other aspects of his body that may not work so well. His body is still, however, unequivocally different. Participation in competitive wheel-chair activities or in the Paralympics is a powerful testimony to physical achievement. The triumph of a successful wheelchair athlete is an image that everyone can commend. But wheelchair sport is not 'real sport'; the Paralympics are not the Olympic Games. While paralysed people may find inspiration in the sporting feats of other people with disabilities, the 'trickle-down' effect may be less than imagined (Hindson & Gidlow 1994), and few able-bodied people would aspire to being in such a position.

The world of disability is different. The bodies of people with disabilities are different. To encourage people with disabilities to imitate the values of the world of able-bodied men is to set them up for failure. A person with a disability may perform 'incredibly well for a disabled person', but a damaged body can never achieve the physical capabilities of a body that is undamaged. While 'good for a paraplegic' may be an important source of self-esteem and pride for many men with these injuries, such praise is constrained by its special category. Like special services in other areas of life, the particularity of the service and thus the activities that occur in such domains are evaluated in the same terms. Such achievements may constrain, rather than liberate, the achiever.

The irony that success in physical rehabilitation may serve to deepen the impact of a disability is a serious cause for concern. More important, though, is the fact that the majority of people who require rehabilitation services are effectively disenfranchised by this focus. People with extensive or progressive losses, or women whose socialisation and gender roles leave them unprepared for physical activities, or unwilling to engage in activities that will further alter the appearance of their bodies, are disadvantaged by this model.

Yet the physical model is a seductive route. The physicality–masculinity connection is central to patriarchy; it is a focus sanc-tioned by the able-bodied world. Continual reaffirmation of the body by comparison with the bodies of others is the substance of men's culture from earliest childhood. Discipline, strength, control, tenacity, endurance and competition are values associated with men's bodies that are understood and shared in society. The notion that competition will bring out the best in us derives from the same source (Clarke & Clarke 1982, p. 83). Would we cease to strive without the incentive of winning? Is the legitimation of public applause the prize we seek in all our endeavours? Is patronising attention better than no attention at all?

A chapter that sets out to explore the implications for reembodiment of the masculinity–physicality connection in formal rehabilitation should foreshadow, but not necessarily explore, alternative areas of rehabilitative potential. Many of the informants had, or have since developed, significant satisfaction in their lives in areas that have little or nothing to do with the physicality of their initial rehabilitative experience. Mary is very interested in cultural things—'music, ballet and that sort of thing'. Sally found music very important during her early days in the unit. Her evaluation of the rehabilitation unit is recorded earlier. She says that during this time

I listened to a lot of music. Probably the best part of the experience was listening to music. That's actually what brought the first movement back. When I was still in the acute hospital one of the nurses brought in all these old tapes. They were Beatles and really old stuff. I am lying there imagining that I am tapping my toes to the music and I notice the sheet moving. I thought, gee, something is moving under there. I got the nurse in and she pulled the sheet back, and I was actually moving my toe! That was the first movement that I got. So I guess music is really a big positive for me—it shuts everything else out.

Pam was 'sport mad and music mad' as a late teenager, and both have been important for her in her subsequent life. Although Pam was unable to perform in musical productions, she was able to continue her connection with the group by taking responsibility for the costumes and make-up. She was also able to develop her considerable talents in singing by joining a choral group. Certainly, Pam also played a considerable amount of sport, 'table tennis being my international sport', and she reached a high level in sports administration.

Pam, like Sally, is quick to recognise that, 'because of my disability, many doors have opened that would never have opened otherwise. My life has taken another direction because of my disability.' Pam's life could have taken another, completely different direction if her musical talents and interests had been given the same focus as her sporting interests in her rehabilitation. The taken-for-granted emphasis on physicality obscures other avenues of rehabilitative potential.

Joy and Tina enjoy wheelchair dancing. While this activity does not enjoy the same privileged position as wheelchair sport in popular imagination, it is not hard to see how much pleasure this could bring people in terms of both exercise and sociability. Peter says: 'I was an artist prior to my accident, however, because of my job I didn't have time to paint. It was a hobby then, whereas now it is my occupation.' Peter now has no hand function at all and must paint with 'a splint attached to my hand to hold a brush and a pencil.' Further development of this pre-existing ability was not raised at all during his time in the unit. Within the scope of this chapter it is sufficient to indicate that many significant avenues of rehabilitative potential exist beyond the penumbra of the prevailing paradigm.

Of course competitive, physical rehabilitation is extremely important for some people with disabilities, despite its restrictive nature. But people who take this route are not only few in number, as discussed earlier, but also represent the 'easiest' rehabilitative challenge. The dimensions of rehabilitation as a whole are defined in terms of these people who appeal to established social values and public altruism, but who also represent the 'easy' part of the broader issue of disability and its rehabilitative response. The rehabilitation enterprise is judged by its 'functional elite': those people who have lost less in physical terms, and who are further advantaged by their masculinity, their physicality and their youth.

Despite the putative power of competition, rehabilitation is not a game. Rehabilitation cannot continue to be shaped by the norms of the physical world to which so few of its clients can aspire. Rehabilitation is about people's lives; it must be concerned with the needs of everyone who seeks its services. By presenting its 'best products' for public scrutiny in this way, rehabilitation diminishes and ignores the lives of many people with a disability. The success of rehabilitation should be judged by how well it deals with its most difficult clients, not by how well it promotes its easiest ones. True rehabilitation for all people with disabilities—men and women, young and old, rich and poor—will involve workers and clients pooling their creative energies to discover avenues for re-embodiment of the whole person in a way that may defy dominant social attitudes about the body. It is undeniable that sport and physical activities provide a context for enjoyment, self-identity and competence, but unless the conditions and ideology of sport are challenged, women, and indeed many men, will continue to operate in a context that compounds their disadvantage.

Finding the impetus to explore the scope and fluidity of broad masculinities and femininities beyond the boundaries of conventional categories of masculinity and femininity will be difficult for workers and disabled people alike. However, it is only by challenging the hegemony of the physicality–masculinity model which has dominated rehabilitation for so long that rehabilitation can be reclaimed as the province of all people with damaged bodies, rather than being just the prerogative of a few.

5 Intimate activities: sexuality

This study explores the interrelationship of the body, the mind and society in the process of making and remaking the body. People come to know their bodies, and to interpret the anatomical and physiological aspects of their bodily systems and endocrine processes, in terms of social categories. Civilised life is achieved by controlling and constraining the body (Turner 1987, p. 98). The young body is trained and educated to embody current social conventions. Civilised in terms of basic physiological functions, the adult body is still enveloped within society. While social life in general depends on controlling and constraining the body, the management of sexuality, in particular, is highly socially regulated (Turner 1987, p. 98). Sexuality, however, is a volatile and anarchic element in civilised society; it has the power to disrupt and subvert social order.

Yet ironically, the ideology of individualism bedevils this topic. Issues associated with sexuality are seen as 'best not spoken about', or as personal problems which should be dealt with at an individual, not a social, level. Emotions such as embarrassment, shame, humiliation and guilt act to reinforce the privacy of such issues and underline their unsuitability for public discourse. The social construction of intimacy extorts a high cost in return for its pleasures. The individual is expected to take responsibility for issues that are often beyond his or her control. Despite the individualisation of these issues, however, private troubles are social issues.

The body is central to sexuality, and sexuality is a major preoccupation of our lives. We need a body in order to be sexual; intimacy depends on the body. Yet paradoxically sexuality, the most intimate aspect of embodiment, is subject to significant control by others. This chapter explores the experience of disrupted sexuality for the embodied self and the processes involved in re-embodiment. Paralysed bodies are disordered bodies in terms of dominant constructions of normality. Although modesty can be a repressive social construction, modesty is also an expression of the freedom to choose that which one wishes to keep private and that which one is happy for others to know about oneself. Privacy, modesty, self-worth, intimacy and sexuality are tied to our ability to take care of our own bodies and to control information about our embodied selves. While the secrecy surrounding issues of sexuality may be an impediment to re-embodiment, dependence on others opens the embodied self to the scrutiny and evaluation of others. Paralysed bodies offer a rare opportunity to witness the implications of unbridled anatomy and physiology, to observe a body that has escaped its social shackles. Paralysed bodies illuminate that which we take for granted. To learn how people who have experienced such catastrophic bodily alterations cope with a non-conformist and vulnerable body provides critical insights into a more general understanding of the body in society.

The reader will find areas of overlap in all of the chapters that contain material from the informant's narratives. This will be especially so in chapters 3 and 5 and to a lesser extent in chapter 6. It is not hard to see that issues concerning the development of relationships must inevitably engage with sexual themes, and that for many of the informants the issues associated with bodily continence will intrude into both these domains. Similarly, fertility and parenting cannot be detached from the themes of either relationships or sexuality, except by an artificial process of separation which would detract from the free flow of the informants' narratives upon which this study is based. I raise this in order to prepare the reader for some repetition of data associated with the interconnected themes in this study.

It is important to begin this analysis of intimacy and bodily disruption with an inventory of the range of bodily losses and changes that the informants may have experienced. In terms of the actual mechanical aspects of sexual function and performance, women with spinal injuries could be seen to fare better than their male counterparts. The paramount factor in this contention is that a spinally injured woman retains her fertility. Menstruation usually ceases at the time of the trauma, but it most often resumes two to three months after the injury (Stewart 1981, p. 347). A paralysed woman can still participate in penile–vaginal intercourse, she can conceive a child in this manner and can produce a healthy baby from her damaged body. The personal and social advantages of these capabilities are immense (Seymour 1989, p. 111). Loss of movement and sensation are, of course, devastating—but in the limited terms of the dominant construction of heterosexuality, a woman's lack of movement and her inability to experience genital pleasure are not of functional importance. Active male: passive female, man's instrument—woman as receptacle is the modus operandi of conventional male–female sexual encounters (Matthews 1984: ch. 7; Rowland 1988, pp. 125–9).

Men with spinal injuries sustain far greater loss in terms of sexual function and ability. Like women, men lose movement and sensation, but since men's role in conventional intercourse is to be the active, initiating partner, their loss of movement may well be more profoundly felt. Men may also lose the ability to obtain an erection and to ejaculate, resulting in greatly impaired fertility (Trieschmann, 1980).

Men with spinal cord damage have two types of erections: reflex and psychogenic. Reflex erections require local contact. They are associated with upper motor neuron spastic injuries, and up to ninety per cent of men with such lesions may have a reflex erection. It is rare for these men to ejaculate. Psychogenic erections occur with lower motor neuron, flaccid lesions. About thirty per cent of men with this impairment have erections. Unlike reflex erections which require local contact, psychogenic erections are the response to cortical activity involving vision and fantasy. Some men with lower motor neuron lesions may have emissions of sperm (Stewart 1981, p. 348).

A man with paralysis from spinal injuries thus has a significant number of losses in relation to sexual activities. In common with a woman with similar spinal damage he has lost movement and sensation. In addition to these losses, however, he has lost the ability to have an erection at will, and therefore his capacity to engage in penile–vaginal intercourse has been jeopardised. Furthermore, since he can no longer ejaculate viable sperm cells into a woman's vagina, he has lost the ability to conceive a child, and is effectively infertile. Much work has been done in this important area of men's sexuality and reproduction in recent years. Technical developments in prosthetics and electro-stimulation may bring hope to some people (Stewart 1981, p. 348), and modern reproductive technologies may present new opportunities for previously impotent and infertile men. Sexuality and fertility, though, have meaning for men that goes far beyond their functional significance. Losses associated with these activities may be profoundly felt.

An incomplete spinal lesion means that some of the spinal nerves have escaped damage, hence the activities supported by these intact nerves remain functional. Although some of the men in this study have incomplete lesions and therefore experience less-predictable loss, for the most part the men with spinal injuries have lost the functions and activities that have been described here. The men's sexuality and reproductive potential have dramatically changed. Loss of bladder and bowel control is also involved in spinal cord damage. Both women and men experience these losses; the implications for management and the impact on embodiment are, however, quite different for men than for women. While relevant to the content of this chapter, issues associated with continence will be discussed more fully in chapter 6.

Although fifteen of the twenty-four informants have experienced injury to their spinal cord, the remaining nine informants have incurred damage from other causes, as discussed in chapter 2. For this reason their losses in relation to sexual activities are less predictable. All have lost considerable degrees of voluntary movement; some live with profound loss. Similarly, all have lost at least some degree of sensation; most of the non-traumatically injured men and women have extensive sensory loss. The fertility of all of the women and most of the men in this group is unimpaired. Although most of these men and women are continent in terms of bladder and bowel function, difficulties with sensation and with mobility confound this advantage.

The dimensions of sexuality extend far beyond the mechanics of sexual performance. Ideas about sexuality, bodily attitudes and experiences and society are critically related. Society influences the ideas, the values, the bodily manifestations and social practices associated with sexuality for men and women. Sexuality is integral to the development and maintenance of the embodied self. Sexuality, then, is a central aspect of re-embodiment after bodily disruption. Dominant constructions of masculinity and femininity may act to further handicap the already disembodied men and women.

Active sexual participation involves finding a partner, or renegotiating the dimensions of a previously established relationship, which may be just as difficult. Attraction and connection, appearance and pairing are essential to the development of a new relationship. Yet the barriers associated with these preliminary activities may pre-empt the possibility of a sexual relationship for people with disabilities. Existing relationships are not exempt either, since one partner must adjust to the new appearance and changed situation of the other partner. To assume that nothing has changed is to ignore the enormous changes that have actually occurred. These preliminaries to sexuality—appearance and relationship development—have been explored in chapter 2 and chapter 3.

It is ironic that despite the fact that a woman will experience less physical loss than a man with spinal injuries, her physical advantage may prove to be an empty blessing in terms of her sexual and reproductive opportunities. Emphasised femininity (Connell 1987, p. 183) is a consistent construction. Youth, specific bodily appearances, shapes and postures are prerequisite, along with particular attitudes and behaviours. Within a specific society the components of this construction are stylised and impoverished (Connell 1987, p. 183); the threshold of tolerance for divergence from the set variables is low. A woman who has experienced severe bodily damage must remake her embodied self within these rigid social categories. Faced with the harsh components of the social construction of a sexual woman, how can a woman reconstitute her damaged self after disease or injury? Society, not clinical losses, may determine her future.

If men's sexuality is symbolised by 'the primacy of the penis' (Lawler 1991, p. 98), the loss of the ability to obtain penile erection at will must be a devastating loss for the men in this study. In terms of 'the phallocentric definition of erotic exchanges which are predicated on a hydraulic notion of the penis and its needs' (Gunew 1987, p. 73) the impact of this loss is immense. Fear that the genital organ may fail to produce a working erection on demand is but one step removed from castration, men's most primal fear. 'Spreading his seed', 'sowing wild oats': distasteful though these phrases must be to many men, they are nevertheless part of male mythology (Connell & Dowsett 1992, p. 56). To be unable to ejaculate, to be unable to spread one's seed, is thus a severe challenge to masculinity. To be denied the pleasures of fathering a child is a profound loss for many men, apart from the strain that infertility must bring to a relationship. Cessation of both genetic and material inheritance is a serious assault to the continuity upon which patriarchy is based. The losses sustained both by the women and the men directly challenge conventional ideas of masculine and feminine sexuality. In no other activity or part of the body is this confrontation so overt. How have the men and women in this study experienced these challenges?

IMPACT OF SEXUAL LOSS

For David, the possibility that he had lost sexual function was the most devastating thought after he was involved in a car accident at the age of fifteen. This fear, in fact, was not realised, as the incompleteness of the lesion spared David his fertility and his sexual function. He now has a six-year-old son. David had 'lost his virginity' about a week before the accident. The significance of this event no doubt projected the issue of sexuality to the forefront of his mind after the injury. Similarly, the first question George asked the surgeon on the night he broke his neck concerned the possibility of sexual loss. Even at seventeen, the loss of fertility was paramount amongst his fears. Ian was twenty when he sustained extensive body paralysis. As a sailor he had experienced a very active sexual life: 'That side of my life was always very important to me.' Ian was able to develop various relationships with staff members during his long stay in a rehabilitation unit. He attributes his successful personal rehabilitation to the self-affirming power of these sexual encounters—'experiences of various kinds, limited one might say'—which occurred early in his institutional stay. Mark was nineteen when he realised that his previous assumptions about sexual practices and fatherhood would not be realised. Although most of the men in the study claim that they were distressed by the spectre, and for many of the men the subsequent reality, of sexual loss, Peter claims that 'too much emphasis is placed on disability and sexuality'. He says that the 'sexual implications never really hit me. I try to play it down because I see other things are important. It is not the most important thing to me.' Although Ron had become sexually active at fifteen or sixteen, some five years before his accident, he claims that 'it wasn't something really important to me'. Now in his early thirties his inability to ejaculate or to have an erection at will is a serious impediment to his desire to develop a relationship and to become a father.

For Joy, injured in a car accident at the age of twenty-two, her loss of ability to experience an orgasm during sexual intercourse is her most serious loss. Sexuality was well incorporated into Frances's sense of self before her illness. She took her sexuality for granted, until severe illness threw her previous complacency into chaos. Mary attributes her successful rehabilitation after the serious physical and sensory losses she sustained in her early thirties to the attentions of a new partner some three years after her accident. Pam was allowed to go home for the weekend at a very early stage of her rehabilitation program after the car accident that caused paralysis of her lower limbs. Pam considers that this was a critical factor in the continuation of her satisfying sexual relationship with her husband. 'We were sleeping in the same bed, and sleeping together after six weeks, so I guess I wasn't really without that part of our marriage.' Although Rosemary is not concerned about her sexuality yet, she can see that this may well become a problem as she becomes older. Rosemary has been paralysed since birth, and is in her early twenties. The relationship between parental expectations and disabled adolescent women's degrees of involvement and success in the heterosexual arena may well be of relevance here (Rousso 1988, p. 139).

No matter what form, practice, context or relationship in which people express their sexuality, sexuality remains an intractable component of embodiment, even if suppressed. Sexuality is a critical component of self-identity. Disruption to the body, no matter how minor, threatens the fragility of the embodied self. The dramatic bodily disruptions experienced by the people in this study confront the conventions associated with sexuality in society. Therefore it is not surprising that the most common assumption about people with extensive bodily damage is that they are asexual (Bogle & Shaul 1981; Bullard & Knight 1981; Campling 1981; Morris 1989). Changes in genital function and in muscle innervation have certainly occurred, but to extrapolate beyond these physical losses seriously exacerbates the damage for the men and women concerned. Genital dysfunction, it seems, simultaneously dismisses all thoughts of carnal and sensual pleasure from people's minds. People with disabilities 'don't do that sort of thing', nor do they 'think about that sort of thing'. Apparently the pleasures that they may have derived from these sorts of things in the past are also expunged from their memory. The physical catastrophe has erased every vestige of sexuality from their embodiment and from their memories.

As Morris, herself disabled, writes: 'Overnight we pass into a state where many people assume we are asexual, often in order to hide embarrassment about the seemingly incongruous idea that such "abnormal" people can have "normal" feelings and relationships' (Morris 1989, p. 80). Although these dismissive assumptions may be comfortable for able-bodied people, they constitute a devastating disenfranchisement for the men and women concerned. The conflation of clinical loss with social discrimination exaggerates the actual damage that has occurred, and seriously threatens sexual eligibility. The physical damage is profound, but it is the meaning that this loss acquires in relation to fixed and rigid social categories of masculinity and femininity that is the real handicap that men and women must bear. Embodiment may be threatened more by the discriminatory attitudes of others than by the actual physical loss.

In an attempt to challenge the assumption of asexuality, Ellen Stohl, an American woman with paraplegia, posed nude for *Playboy* magazine (Hume 1990, p. 1). An Australian woman with a disability later posed for a similar magazine (Lonsdale 1990, p. 7). Many women would consider that such exposure constitutes an act of betrayal. For a woman with a disability to display herself in this way compounds the betrayal: she betrays both her sex and the disability movement which has identified prejudice based on appearance as the major source of discrimination for people with disabilities. Ironically, these acts may also be seen as a symbol of the ultimate emancipation of women with disabilities: the right to be perceived as a sex object and accordingly enshrined on the altar to male sexual fantasy, the *Playboy* centrefold (Hume 1990, p. 1).

So although such acts reinforce the narrow, confining view of women's bodies and sexuality that dominates popular culture, they could also be seen as a courageous assertion of bodily difference. In displaying their bodies in this way the women defy the usual impoverished and confining representations of women with disabilities and celebrate the integrity of their embodiment, a task similar to that undertaken by Hevey (1992) and Spence (1986) with a camera.

PROFESSIONAL NEGLECT OF SEXUAL ISSUES

The informants in this study repeatedly condemn health workers in institutional and professional situations for their neglect of sexual issues, or for the sexism embedded in their advice on the rare occasions that it is given. Rehabilitative attention focuses on issues associated with men's bodies, and is seldom concerned with women's bodies. The literature on spinal cord injury is dominated by male problems of erection, orgasm and fertility; female sexuality is dismissed (Deegan 1985, p. 48; Fine & Asch 1988, p. 3; Lonsdale 1990, p. 8). The problems involved in men's re-embodiment are profound, but so are the less dramatic, but equally important issues associated with sexuality as a component of women's re-embodiment. It is not sufficient to excuse this bias on the basis of the statistical preponderance of men with spinal cord injuries. Understanding the differential treatment of men and women requires a thorough analysis of rehabilitation as a practice embedded within the profession of medicine, and the physical, mechanical and masculine domination of that paradigm. More critically, this bias reflects the central meaning of man's penis and man's seed as both the symbolic potency and the pragmatic reality of hegemonic masculinity.

Alister was married and had two sons at the time of the accident that caused his quadriplegia. He claims that no one in the rehabilitation unit talked with him about his sexual loss or about his future sexual possibilities. However, he claims that 'I was always an individual, and I wanted to go out on my own and get my own counsel.' Sexuality was 'never discussed' during Bob's rehabilitation about fifteen years ago. 'The whole sexuality issue was very important to me, there were all these pipes and tubes coming out of me. I wondered what was going on. I kept asking questions about having children, and not getting a lot of answers.' Bob claims that he asked everybody about this issue, 'nursing staff, doctors and other patients, but the best information came from other patients'. During this time he came to the understanding that he was infertile. 'For about four years I just thought that I couldn't have children, then I met this lady and I could ejaculate and I had two kids.'

The fact that James could not give me any examples of attempts by professional workers to discuss his own sexuality with him is a sad reflection of the difficulty such workers have in dealing with people who have been damaged since birth, or who have progressively disabling conditions. James contends that

> the only real examples I have are other's experiences. One really disabled person inquired about the sexual options available to him through his doctor during the time he was at [names rehabilitation unit]. The solution was simply to give him a book called Sexual Options for Paras and Quads, and indicate that he would like it back in a week. To me that was not therapy. Thank God things have changed a bit since those days. The problem is that those professionals up there regard sexuality as something that should not be encouraged, in fact it should be discouraged, avoided and distracted from and this is why basketball was encouraged as it takes away energy.

When asked about how he learned about the extent and implications of his sexual loss Ken claims that 'I asked and I never really got a satisfactory answer. Ultimately how I found out about my post-disability sexuality was just with my girlfriend and myself.' Although Ken realised that the issues of sexual function can be complex, especially in relation to incomplete lesions, he resents the fact he was always 'the instigator of any information, no one volunteered any information. I never got any satisfactory information while I was in hospital.'

The 'basketball cure' was also offered to Mark as a solution to his distress about his sexual loss:

> When word got around that I was a bit concerned about all this they lined me up to see the urologist. There he was sitting on the other side of the desk with his pin-striped suit on, looking very suave. He said 'How old are you?'. I think I said that I was twenty. He said, 'Oh, look that's really young and I believe you play basketball. Look, I reckon you should get into the basketball, you're young, you've got plenty of time to work things out, just take your mind off it and go out and play basketball'. So, no wonder I played basketball!

Jenny felt that she couldn't talk to anyone about her future sexual possibilities. Some time later she went to an 'alternative medicine doctor', about another problem. 'The doctor said "What do most women feel on intercourse anyway? A lot of it is about closeness and sense of involvement, as distinct from the physical sensation of intercourse for women". And that was, I think, the first step, the first little seeds for me feeling that I didn't have to perceive it as my problem.'

Pam's injury occurred many years ago. No one talked with her about her sexuality while she was in the unit, nor was she given advice about the maintenance of her sexual relationship with her husband. Joy was also distressed about the lack of attention to this critical aspect of embodiment during her time in the rehabilitation unit much more recently.

I was told to talk to the social worker. What could she offer me? She is an able-bodied woman. She knows nothing. There is some lady out there you can talk to, she is a woman in a wheelchair, but she charges ten dollars an hour to come to talk to you. There is no way I am paying that. It should be offered to you there at the rehabilitation unit.

Joy's experiences are quite recent; Pam's and Joy's experiences serve to illustrate how little things have changed in relation to attention to women's sexuality in the quarter of a century that has elapsed between the post-injury rehabilitation of these two women.

The attitudes of staff to the sexuality of people with damaged bodies who must spend a large part of their lives in residential accommodation is clearly based on the assumption of asexuality discussed before, and is particularly destructive. Tina described how difficult it was to develop any sort of personal relationship in such settings. The issue of privacy is particularly difficult. She describes an incident between two residents who had a relationship, but had nowhere to go to express their feelings toward each other: 'Because there was no privacy they would touch each other in the corridor. One nurse said to me, "So-and-so hasn't got knickers on today. I know why—so that so-and-so can touch her". I said, "Well you can go home can't you, you've got your boyfriend at home?" She just shut up after that.' Alison, like Tina, has spent a large part of her life in an institution. She says: 'I would never recommend anyone in an institution to try to make a relationship work because it doesn't. Everyone interferes; everyone just wanted to have their say.' Alison is now very happily married, she lives in a suburban house with her husband and together they run a successful business.

Despite their efforts to obtain professional advice about the extent and implications of their losses, most people picked up clues about their sexual futures incidentally, and from a variety of informal sources. In the early days of his rehabilitation, David wore a leg bag for urinary drainage. He can remember asking one of the sisters: '"What is that white stuff at the bottom of the bag?" She said, "That's sperm", and I said, "Can I still do it?" She said, "You'll get odd reactions like that all the time", and that was about it. Nothing related to me at all sexually out there. It affected me pretty badly, I think, being a fifteen-year-old especially.' Seventeen-year-old George showed similar anxiety about sexual loss. The first question he asked the surgeon on the night he broke his neck concerned this issue. 'I shocked the surgeon. He gave me a big, churchy lecture on that one.' Although he was extremely anxious about his sexuality, Bob remembers picking up clues from other people along the lines of 'don't worry about this, just get yourself mobile'. He claims that these messages that he should not be concerned with sexual matters were the reason that he 'put my own sexuality on hold for a while'.

Sally was a nurse at the time of her accident, so many of the aspects of sexual function that were mysterious to many of the other men and women were already known to her. Nevertheless, Sally laments the fact that fifteen years ago there was no professional guidance for the men or women with disabilities on 'what to expect from life, what to expect sexually, or what to expect emotionally and socially with friends and family'. Sally claims to feel particularly sorry for the men. When asked to explain this statement she says: 'As a woman, it doesn't change me. A guy may be impotent. He has to re-learn to use himself in different ways and do those sorts of things that guys, with their classic male ego, rely on for their sexual status. I really felt for a lot of guys.' Sally's concern for spinally injured men is kindly motivated, but it is clear that her thinking is bound to an assumption of female sexual passivity implicit in conventional heterosexuality. Loss of movement and sensation seem nothing when compared with a man's loss of control over penile erection.

Ellie Becker, herself a paraplegic, bemoans the lack of attention to issues associated with the sexuality of spinally injured women. Information, she claims, is almost exclusively male focused. If women are mentioned at all, it is in relation to their child-bearing capacities. One must assume, she suggests, that the minimisation of women's adjustment difficulties occurs because a woman does not have to contend with the horrific problems associated with a malfunctioning 'magic wand' (Becker 1978, p. vii). Such perspectives not only are 'extremely insensitive to the richly endowed and magnificently complex area of female sexuality', but also perpetuate highly stereotypic and narrow ideas of both male and female sexual potentiality. Becker concludes her book with the hope that the insights of the informants in her study will inspire awareness of the need for 'thorough,

understanding sexual counseling and complete sexual information'
(1978, p. 259).

Becker's wish has not been realised. Today, nearly twenty years
later, sexuality is still a profound issue for both men and women
with severe bodily paralyses. Reproductive issues for women and the
mechanical aspects of male erection, ejaculation and sperm production dominate the literature. These concerns mimic the major tenets
of hegemonic sexuality under patriarchy. Rigid sex roles imprison
men's and women's bodies; traditional categories may seriously
impede re-embodiment after serious bodily disruption. A catastrophe
may offer a person the opportunity to increase the richness of sexual
expression and experience. Yet active male, passive female is the
choreography of heterosexual interrelationships implicit in the
assumptions underlying modern rehabilitation. Sexuality, as distinct
from the mechanics of sexual performance, remains obscured in
contemporary rehabilitation programs.

SEXUAL EXPERIENCES

Paraplegia and quadriplegia are masculine conditions. This does not
mean that women do not acquire these conditions, as the women in
this study clearly prove. In our society, men are encouraged to engage
in the kinds of activities that put the spinal cord, as well as many
other parts of the body, at risk. The thrill of contact sports and
some, typically male, leisure activities, is engendered because these
activities challenge the body. Challenging the body and competing
with other men in contests of bodily strength and endurance have
been central to male identity, at least since the days of Odysseus.
These issues have been explored extensively in chapter 4. Drinking
alcohol and travelling in fast cars—one or the other, or the dangerous
combination of the two—are also critical tenets of hegemonic masculinity, a masculinity most powerfully expressed in young bodies.
Not only are the majority of the clients of spinal injuries rehabilitation units male, but they are also young (Seymour 1989, p. 62).

Women nursing men back to health after severe injury or sickness
is a common theme in literature and popular culture. The weakness
and dependence of the man's body enables the woman to take a
more active role in the male–female relationship (Coward 1984,
p. 195). Female nurse–male patient interactions violate the conventions of social life (Lawler 1991, ch. 9). Physical vulnerability, nudity,
dependence, sexuality, gratitude, embarrassment and power create
highly volatile situations where the suspension of normality predisposes unusual behaviours and expectations. Although the
management of such situations is the subject of considerable

professional concern (Emerson 1973, p. 358; Lawler 1991), the potential for anarchy is always present. The youth and maleness of the client group in a spinal injuries unit contrasts with the overwhelming femaleness of the staff. Physiotherapists, occupational therapists and nurses are likely to be female. These professional workers spend a lot of time each day with the clients; treatments extend over many months in the 'encompassing world of the patient' (Seymour 1989, p. 88). Pringle's exploration of 'organisational sexuality', the interweaving of sexuality in the routine labour processes of bosses and secretaries, resembles aspects of gendered staff and client interrelationships in rehabilitation units (Pringle 1988). It is not hard to see how intimate relationships can develop in such situations. Many examples of staff–client relationships have been documented already in chapter 3. Professional worker–patient relationships are clearly more than just the stuff of fiction.

The vulnerability of people with intellectual disability to abuse is well documented in the literature (Abdilla 1992; Breckenridge & Carmody 1992, Finger 1985) but poorly addressed in practice. People who have experienced catastrophic physical losses are also vulnerable to abuse (Lonsdale 1990, p. 72). These people are entirely dependent on others for a considerable time, some for ever. Other people have access to the paralysed person's body in ways that would be quite unacceptable in everyday life. Not only are paralysed people severely limited in the ways that they can protect their body from the scrutiny of others, but they are unable to move to avoid unpleasant encounters. The power differential between the carer and the recipient of care compounds the vulnerability associated with restricted mobility. The survival of the paralysed person depends on the goodwill of other people, either in a professional or paid capacity, or within the bounds of the family or neighbourhood at least initially, if not for the rest of the person's life. Such dependency on others heightens the vulnerability of such people to physical, sexual, psychological and domestic abuse.

Formal hospital policies that forbid staff to fraternise with patients obviously reflect this concern. Bob claims that in his experience, 'I haven't seen anyone taken for a ride'. No doubt though, emotional pain and further damage to an already fragile self-identity may be associated with such practices. The discursive opportunities, contradictory realities and rich ambiguities of staff–client interrelationships, however, are powerful elements in the reflexive project of re-embodiment. For some people, the overwhelming self-affirming potential of these early experiments with sexuality must justify their continuance, covert and potentially dangerous though they may be.

A person's previous sexual experience plays a crucial role in their embodiment, and in the range of reconstitutive resources that he or she is able to bring to the task of re-embodiment. Many of the men and women who had experienced the sudden losses associated with spinal injuries or paralysing infections were able to draw on the past to find strategies for the reflexive project of the self (Giddens 1991, p. 5).

Frances's relationship with her husband had been constructed on the basis of a very physically dominant self-image. This was the way her husband saw her; this was the way she viewed herself:

> *He was very conscious of physical appearance, and for me not to be this physically perfect being that he thought he had chosen to be his partner was very distressing for him. He could never say to me 'Well it doesn't matter what you look like, you are still OK'. His problem was that he wanted to make me well, he saw it as a sense of failure that he couldn't.*

Relationships since the breakup of her marriage have affirmed just those aspects of her sexual identity that she felt that she had lost in her disease. Rather than wishing that her body was 'perfect', new partners

> *have been able to talk about my body and say that they loved me, admired me, whatever—and they'll say it is not only because your face is beautiful, but I love those bits of you that don't work so well, that aren't what you want them to be. They don't push these issues aside, they raise them. It is the most incredible experience for affirming someone.*

Ian had been a sailor when he acquired the virus that was to cause such extensive damage to his body: 'Being at sea, of course, I had a lot of opportunity for a very active life sexually. So to have all of that cut off not only physically, but also mentally reduced, was a particularly devastating assault on my psyche. Those women staff members restored the possibility to me that this need not stop.' The physical dimensions of a sexual body were also an important component of Joy's embodiment before her accident. At seventeen, and living in another State she

> *got paid seventy dollars an hour for doing photographic model- ling. It was all nude, but I wouldn't do an open leg shot for anybody. I used to get men offering me more money to do this, but that is distasteful. A woman's body is the most beautiful thing that God invented, apart from nature itself. It is there to be appreciated and not neglected and just used for sex and that is all.*

Ken's self-confidence with past sexual relationships gave him the confidence to re-embody his sexuality as a paraplegic:

I mean I've always been pretty arrogant anyway, but I basically never had any problems with women. I was a bit of a chauvinist, and I guess I retained some of those values to some extent. Women were there for me and for my convenience, and yeah, so that's changed—but that's part of growing up, rather than having a disability. I do think that the disability has impacted on my maturity and behaviour in a lot of different ways, and in that context, I think that it has been a positive thing.

However, many of the informants did not have a legacy of ideas and experiences associated with their own sexuality. The management of their disability by others had effectively disqualified these men and women from sexual participation since childhood. James, Alison and Tina, unlike the previous men and women, did not have the opportunity to develop a strong, sexual aspect to their embodiment. The serious nature of the conditions these people have necessitated institutional living from a relatively early age. The alleged need to regulate life in such bureaucratic situations, coupled with lack of privacy and assumptions of asexuality meant that these people had little opportunity to transcend the 'problem' of their disordered bodies.

Despite these impediments, Alison developed her first serious relationship when she was about eighteen years old. This relationship lasted for eight years, but although it was 'very, very close', it never became a physical relationship. Later Alison became engaged to a young man in the institution. 'We had a physical relationship and we decided that we were going to get engaged and get married.' However Alison's friend broke off the engagement. Despite these two painful episodes, Alison has been married for the last five or six years, and says that she is very happy.

Although James would love to have an intimate relationship, so far he has been unable to establish an on-going relationship. Tina attributes her difficulties in finding a sexual partner to the rigidity of gender stereotypes. 'Because women are usually the carers men tend to think, "Oh my God, I am going to have to look after this woman for the rest of my life".' In their kindness and support of her, Tina's parents may also have been an impediment to the development of aspects of their daughter's sexuality. Discussion of such issues would be 'out of the question because of their cultural and religious background'. Tina's closeness to her parents would not encourage her to offend their beliefs. That these three people— Alison, James and Tina—lead interesting and productive lives in the community today is testimony to their personal resilience and their strength in overcoming the obstacles placed in their way by the professional and bureaucratic policies of the past.

In the absence of satisfactory discussion or advice from professional sources, most people claim that they had no recourse but to discover the extent and implications of their sexual loss by 'trying it out'. While this method may well make sense in the long run, such experimentation requires great bravery on the part of people who have already suffered a devastating challenge to their self-identity. Sexuality involves vulnerability and uncertainty about body appearance and performance. Most people feel insecure about intimate exposure: they fear being evaluated poorly by those they most wish to please. People develop protective behaviours and defensive strategies to insulate their self-identity against the continual risk of rejection. But it is this element of emotional risk-taking that invests sexual activities with such enormous emotional, physical and social significance. Sexual intercourse is the ultimate act of emotional and physical exposure. Stripped of outer artifice, the body stands bare and alone. The thrill of sexual encounters is increased by this ambient danger and risk.

Sexuality is felt as the stirring of bodily passion, but sexuality is also a product of the learned features of sexual ideology in a particular social context at a particular historical time. The man or woman with a disability has built up a sexual identity of himself or herself in the able-bodied world where sexual stereotypes are strongly articulated. Films, television, pub and sport cultures continually reinforce a consistent image of hegemonic male sexuality. Thrust, strength, force, initiation, movement, power and dominance are critical tenets of this image. Feminine sexuality is similarly encapsulated in clearly recognisable stereotypes, discussed in chapters 2 and 3. Not only are damaged bodies no longer capable of feeling or reacting to stimuli in the same way, but the person's embodied sexuality, built up over many years, is no longer appropriate. The person's previous understandings about the body, its attractiveness to others, and preferred modes of sexual activity must be negated. To continue to pursue the assumptions and practices of the past will perpetuate the chaos and exacerbate the pain. But difficult though it may be to transcend the past, it is infinitely more difficult to challenge social categories in relation to masculine and feminine sexuality. And it is this task that these men and women must face.

David considered that he was luckier than many men because he could still have an erection: 'I knew I could ejaculate, and feel reasonably good. I knew that I had all the physical capabilities, it's just a matter of trying the different methods as far as penetration is concerned. Some of the experiences I had earlier on, before I met

my wife, were very funny. Practice makes perfect.' Despite his
seeming nonchalance about his sexual re-embodiment, David admits
that 'in the back of my mind I did fear a loss of sexuality'. In
common with many of the other spinally injured men, David had
no difficulty in finding female partners to help him explore his new
sexual potential:

> *I didn't have any shortage of partners to go out with, there were
> heaps of people, we had an endless supply, they were always keen
> to go out with you. Some girls really like to go out with guys
> in wheelchairs—whether they feel secure or its something very
> different. Relating to some of the experiences I've had with
> women, I think they find it quite sexually intriguing.*

David goes on to say:

> *It may seem strange, but in a sexual sense I am glad that I am
> a paraplegic. Although I have limited sensation in my penis
> compared to before I was a paraplegic, I can still have an orgasm,
> and ejaculate, but because I have not so much of a sense of relief
> after orgasm, I maintain an erection for ages. It has been a big
> advantage to me. I have also got very slight hips and not much
> weight in my legs, and I am obviously very strong here* [indicating
> the upper chest], *so as far as the continuous thrusting of inter-
> course is concerned, I can go on and on because it is not much
> effort for me. Obviously they enjoy it most of the time.*

Joy also talks about the ultimate masculine fantasy, the priapic
penis. She talks about the short sexual relationship she had with a
fellow paraplegic: 'Two paraplegics in bed together! That's funny.
It's fun, it really is!' She claims that 'there were no problems, apart
from not being able to feel. But we still had fun. We still got pleasure
out of it. We still made love and had sex. But it's fun because the
male paraplegics use a needle to give them an erection. Their penis
stays up for about three or four hours, so there is no problem of
ever losing that.'

In exploring new relationships after the breakup of her marriage
Frances says: 'Displaying myself in a new sexual relationship has
been pretty terrifying, acceptance of my new body by others has
been really critical.' Frances contends that such affirmation was
central to her rehabilitation. By such means Frances was able to
incorporate her disordered body and her damaged self-identity into
a vital new re-embodied sexuality. Although the rewards are immense
for people who are able to repossess their intimate bodies in this
way, the risks of failure are, similarly, immense. Such vulnerability

can lead to despair, but it can also constitute a significant core around which re-embodiment is forged. Many people who are already coping with the enormous burden of bodily disruption may be unwilling to expose their bodies to further evaluation by others. In view of the dangers associated with such situations, the reluctance these people express is entirely understandable. Yet emotional risk-taking removes the person from the protective haven of patient status and propels him or her into the real world of satisfactions and sorrows, the world of intimate and emotional relationships (Seymour 1989, p. 110).

Remnants of conventional romance and courtship continue to impoverish women's sexuality. In waiting to be pursued by a man, women allow others to assume responsibility for their desires (Coward 1984, p. 194). Rosemary, paralysed since birth and now in her early twenties, has not had a boyfriend, but she says: 'I want a boyfriend one day, but I will just have to wait until the right one comes along'. Although she admits to 'a little concern about the sexuality part', she claims 'I suppose I will worry about it later on in life'. When asked if there was anything that she was doing to prepare herself for this she said: 'No, I had sex education classes in high school, I think things will just come naturally. I don't want to read books to find out about life.' Bridget is about the same age as Rosemary, but unlike Rosemary she 'really misses being with the friends she was at school with in the country'. She also misses doing 'the things that people my age do—going out with boyfriends and in groups'. She feels that 'most boys in my age group are immature, they don't know how to approach someone in a wheelchair'. Clearly there are many other aspects of severe bodily disruption beside sexuality itself that may pre-empt the possibility of embarking on a sexual relationship, many of which have been discussed in chapter 3.

Pam, too, felt that 'things just come naturally'. She says that her husband 'just coped with her changed body without ever a comment being made'. Although Pam has lost all movement and sensation below the waist, the fact that she could still give pleasure to her husband and still have a child was extremely significant. Pam claims that she didn't have any discussion with, and certainly received no advice from, any one in the rehabilitation unit about her sexual prospects. On the other hand Pam says: 'I can't remember there being a major problem other than me thinking that this is unfair on my husband, but we gradually learned to overcome that. I never sat there and said this isn't fair on you because we just didn't do that. We just got on with it and coped.'

Pam's ability to deal with extremely difficult situations is most admirable. It is not hard to see, however, how conventional ideas of femininity played out in her coping strategies. Her own significant losses in terms of sexual pleasures and performance are subsumed by the fact that her husband's needs can still be satisfied. Pam commends her husband for 'never commenting that any change had occurred'. It seemed not to have occurred to her that she needed acknowledgment of just how much her enjoyment of her sexual body had been destroyed by the accident. Similarly, the fact that she could still have a child, despite the fact that she was faced with the formidable task of bringing up three young children while in a wheelchair, was extremely important. Motherhood, a critical tenet of conventional femininity, was still available to her. Rosemary's ideas also derive from similar cultural presentations about male–female relationships. The 'one day my prince will come and everything will be wonderful' school of male–female interrelationships (Gilbert & Taylor 1991, p. 78) does little to prepare young people for the realities of relationships. Rosemary, and people with similar bodily damage, are particularly vulnerable.

Joy had her first sexual encounter after her accident soon after leaving the rehabilitation unit. She was pleased to acknowledge this important rehabilitative rite of passage: 'When I arrived at the gym next morning I said, "I got laid last night!" I didn't know what to expect, but I knew that I wouldn't be able to feel anything, so I wasn't feeling really upset. It was really important to have sex again. I was rapt that I had.' Although Joy had enjoyed many sexual relationships before her accident, she too is pleased that she can give her partner pleasure. In contrast to some of the other women, however, she is also concerned about her own enjoyment of sexual activities:

> If I am having sex, it gives me pleasure to know that my partner is getting pleasure. I have lost feeling from just above my belly button. Having sex for me is very frustrating. I still get stimulation through my breast to my clitoris, as before, which is good, but as far as feeling sex through my vagina—there is not much there. It is very frustrating. I haven't had an orgasm for three years. It is part of your life which you lose, which people take for granted. Before I never used to worry about my breast or my neck being touched or bitten or anything like that, now it is all I have really got to focus on. Before I used to hop right into it—enjoy the pleasure of sex, orgasm and stuff—whereas now it is much different.

Early sexual encounters can be extremely damaging for men and women with severe disembodiment. Knowing that you will not be able to feel the pleasure of sexual activity is one thing; actually experiencing what it feels like not to feel is another. The confidence and satisfaction gained in achieving competence in the practical tasks of rehabilitation can be dashed by the realisation that sexuality will never be experienced in the same way again. For some people such a realisation is the final straw in the enormity of their bodily catastrophe. To be restricted in movement and changed in appearance, to be unable to take one's bladder or bowel for granted; as if these losses were not enough to bear, one is also unable to enjoy the pleasures of one's own body or to share the joy and comfort of intimacy with others. Not surprisingly many people relegate their sexuality to the 'back burner' until they feel strong enough to cope with such a dangerous and risk-filled area of their embodied selves.

For many people, transcending the narrow dimensions of conventional masculine and feminine sexuality may be more difficult than overcoming the physical impediments that have occurred. Yet the extent of the losses may offer others the opportunity to address the private, unexamined relationship between their sexuality and embodiment, often for the first time. Such confrontation can lead to exciting new pleasures, to rich, expansive sexualities freed from the confining power of conventional sex roles and relationships. Robert Lenz, who has quadriplegia from a spinal cord injury, is not part of my study, but his insights are relevant here:

> I'm a much better lover now than I ever was before. There are a lot of reasons for that, but one of the biggest is that I'm more relaxed. I don't have a list of do's and don'ts, a timetable or a proper sequence of moves to follow, or the need to 'give' my partner an orgasm every time we make love. Sex isn't just orgasm for me; it's pleasuring, playing, laughing and sharing (Lenz & Chaves 1981, p. 67).

Masturbation has long been seen as a disreputable activity undertaken by children and other 'uncivilised' people (Connell & Dowsett 1992, p. 108). Research studies and surveys in recent years have revealed that contrary to the myth, many people engage in self-stimulation throughout their lives. Yet taboo and prohibition persist about this activity. The paramount role of sexuality in full re-embodiment is undeniable, yet since the body can become the site of pain, embarrassment, uncertainty, fear, guilt and isolation, it is not hard to see how many men and women come to see their body as an enemy (Bogle & Shaul 1981, p. 92). Masturbation may be an extremely important avenue for reclaiming the body, for re-embodying the damage and arousing new sites of pleasure. Apart from its importance in self-knowledge and bodily acceptance, masturbation provides the means for sexuality to be personal and not just 'the privilege of partnership' (Becker 1978, p. 108).

Conventionally, sexual excitement for women arises from

stimulation of the genitals and the breasts. Forced to seek new sources of erotic pleasure, women with paralysed bodies may discover that parts of the body that would not usually have been considered sensual may become sites of intense sexual gratification. By experimenting with various forms of sexual expression and evoking new sensual inputs, many men and women who cannot feel the lower parts of their bodies may discover new erogenous zones. Some women claim that through stimulation of the nipples strong sensation is evoked in the clitoris; in some instances this sensation is as strong as if the clitoris was being stimulated directly. Some women achieve orgasm in this way (Becker 1978, p. 11). This avenue is not available to women with quadriplegia or more extensive paralysis. Moreover, apart from masturbation, such experimentation depends on a willing and a caring partner who is able to transcend social conventions about what men do and how women should respond, as well as his or her own past experiences and practices to learn new ways of giving and receiving pleasure. Access to such ideal partners cannot be taken for granted.

Unlike Frances, Joy has found that many of the men she has encountered since her accident are unable to acknowledge her bodily losses or to help her experiment with new ways of achieving pleasure. Joy says: 'If they are not interested in asking, I am not going to tell them because they don't care how I feel. They are just interested in getting their rocks off and that's it. I won't let the relationship go on any further. If they care enough about me, they will ask and we will try different things.'

Pam claims that the quality of her relationship with her husband persisted because she was able to go home at weekends from a very early stage of her rehabilitation program. Maintaining an existing relationship was more difficult for those men and women who were not able to leave the institution so soon. For Bob 'it was going from seeing the lady every night and day of the week to maybe once a week when she could come down from the country town about 100 kilometres away'. Privacy in an institution is always a difficult issue (Seymour 1989, p. 79). It was a major issue for Bob. 'You like to have a kiss and a cuddle but you never knew whether someone was going to walk in the door. It was almost impossible to continue an intimate relationship with your partner while in the institution.' Sally and her partner did not participate in their former sexual relationship while Sally was in the institution: 'I just was not interested, and he more or less said that I was going through rehabilitation, and really, he was just a visitor. That was the way I chose it to be. Whether he was interested or not, I really don't care. Sex was the last thing on my mind.'

Sally's bravado, though, may well hide her disappointment at the realisation that her 'comfortable relationship', though satisfactory in good times, was not going to survive the considerable changes in her body and in her life. However, acknowledgment of on-going sexuality was a crucial factor in personal rehabilitation for many of the other informants. Frances's husband was able to spend time with her while she was in intensive care. 'One thing which he did which was wonderful, and I would regard as almost out of character for him, was when I was in intensive care and I was lying naked most of the time, he put his hand under the sheet and stroked my breast.' For Frances, this was an immensely important act of affirmation at a time of enormous chaos. Like Pam, Jenny had been able to go home on weekend leave quite soon after the injury. Speaking about her partner, Jenny says:

> I don't remember being touched a lot. I can remember feeling that I needed to. We never had intercourse again. He couldn't . . . and that caused me pain because I was looking for that acceptance. What happened was that we just got into a whole sexuality spiral around that issue. It ended up with him finding erections more difficult or not coming to a climax because there would be this barrier. Later he told me that he just felt this incredible pressure from me to perform and he saw it as a real performance demand. And I wasn't really wanting continuous intercourse, I needed somehow to be given a sense of returning to normal femininity.

FERTILITY

Discussing the changes that occur to the individual body in pregnancy Scarry describes the 'awe-inspiring' capacity of the body 'not simply to persist in its existence [. . .] but to re-assert and replicate its aliveness [. . .] to achieve greater and greater presence'. She suggests that we may undervalue the enormity of this bodily feat 'because we now live at a time when the growth of populations is simply assumed' (Scarry 1985, p. 192).

A basic expectation of most people is that they will be able to have children. Notions of bodily integrity and wholeness are closely tied to fertility. Ancient customs involving the patronymic and patrimony depend on the passage of genetic material from father to son. Concern for the continuation of family name and fortunes, though not so overt, is still important today. Having children confers immortality; after death you live on through your children. Not only can you bequest your accumulation of material possessions to your children, but the memories and meanings constructed throughout your life survive in the children's lives and in the lives of their children.

Childlessness evokes pity. Most women become mothers; those who don't must contend with the notion that adulthood is not achieved without motherhood (Oakley 1986, p.1). Even today, people feel the need to explain why they have not produced children (Lewis 1986). Such people must deal with other people's presumptions that their old age will be lonely, and their thinly veiled implications that life without children is meaningless. In many societies, childlessness is associated with sin, particularly sexual sin. 'If children are the gift of God, the lack of them is God's punishment' (Greer 1984, p. 51).

Paradoxically, contraception is a major preoccupation of people's lives (Greer 1984, p. 34). Yet despite the energy with which we continue to suppress fertility, infertility is a tragedy for many men and women. Infertility is also big business (Rowland 1988, p. 166). Specialties devoted to in-vitro fertilisation and associated techniques are high-prestige areas within medicine, and involve enormous costs, both personal and financial. Yet Rowland claims it is a 'false promise and a failed technology'. The success rate for live births in Australia is between five and ten per cent, in some States as low as four per cent (Rowland 1988, p. 168). Having children is clearly so important that couples, particularly women, will subject themselves to the dangers (Rowland 1988, p. 167) and emotional pain (Bowe 1987, p. 150) of these technologies which offer such low odds for success. Reproduction may offer a possibility of transcending the damaged body, yet the diminished ability of people in this study to have children may compound the tragedy.

In terms of the bodily losses that are the concern of this study, it is possible for all of the women to conceive and give birth to a child. The potentiality and for some, the actuality, of child bearing are clearly of considerable significance. Frances, Mary and Pam each had three children at the time of their bodily crisis. Robyn and Ruth have lived with their bodily conditions all their lives. These two women have each had one child. Jenny, paralysed from the waist down, had a baby last year. The other six women have not had children, though each claims that she would like to. Clearly, there are many issues beyond the pragmatics of fertility that impede these women in having children, many of which have been discussed in the preceding chapters. Yet conception, child bearing and the birth of a baby out of a body that has failed to conform to the desires and wishes of the woman in so many other respects, must seem like a miracle.

Although men with spinal injury fare much less well than their female counterparts with the same level of injury in terms of conventional sexual performance and fertility, again the pragmatics of sexuality and reproduction are only a part of the story. Sexuality and fatherhood are undoubtedly critical to masculinity (Connell 1983), yet many other issues complicate the more technical aspects of these bodily activities. Alister had two sons at the time of his accident, and Bob's partner was pregnant with their child when he became paralysed. George, James, Mark, Peter, Ron and Ken have not had a child, though Ken has two stepchildren. Ian's fertility was left intact by the virus that caused such extensive damage to the rest of his body; he has fathered four children since this time. Similarly, Gerald's fertility was untouched by the source of his bodily loss, and he too has had a child. The incompleteness of Anthony's and David's spinal lesions has meant that these two men have been able to have a child, though not without an enormous amount of intervention in Anthony's case.

Even at fifteen, the possibility that he had lost sexual function was the most devastating issue for David: 'I started asking questions about three days after I woke up'. Mark was similarly distressed by this possibility. He claims that he also 'recognised very early that my sexual functioning had changed. What happened for me was a real sense of loss of my masculinity, my sexual identity.' Mark goes on to say: 'One of my early experiences was of losing sensation. I could get erections, I got erections while having penile cleaning. I used to masturbate a lot before I had my accident. I tried this masturbation thing again, and nothing happened—no ejaculation, no orgasm. It was very distressing because I used to enjoy that.' Mark also realised the implications of this for his fertility. He says he thought, 'Oh no! this was it—no genetic line . . . and so there it goes, no kids'. Even at nineteen he claims that the whole implication of this loss was clear to him: 'This seemed to be very important at the time—I sort of gave up on masturbating from there on for quite a while, in fact for many years—it's crazy, isn't it?'

Ron would like to be a father. He hopes that if his current relationship develops as he hopes, he 'would like to look into it'. Although Ken now has two stepchildren, he would dearly love to have a child of his own. He realises that the situation is often complex with incomplete lesions such as his own, but he resents the fact that he has been given so little opportunity to discuss this important issue with professional people. Ken goes on to say:

Even now [three years after his accident], *I'm going through a process where I'm trying to find out whether I'm fertile or not. I can have an erection at will and I ejaculate sometimes, but not always. What we've discovered is that there are absolutely no sperm in that. We have also discovered that one of my tubes is*

retrograde, and the other is blocked. So I am going through a
series of tests to establish this.

Although Anthony had not had a child at the time we first spoke,
he has subsequently fathered a daughter. Anthony's incomplete quadriplegia has made this an extremely complicated procedure. Anthony
and his wife Kate tried a range of strategies to provoke fertility.
Treatment spread over many years and at various stages included
daily visits to hospital for blood tests and for hormonal injections
to increase fertility, techniques such as electro-ejaculation, artificial
insemination under general anaesthesia and many other measures to
stimulate conception (O'Brien 1992, p. 17). Despite the discomfort,
humiliation, disruption and disappointment that Anthony and Kate
associate with the program (O'Brien 1992, p. 17), it is clear that
they were prepared to endure these distressing experiences in order
to have a child.

Jenny's experience involving a man she felt was attracted to her
because he felt she was less threatening has been documented in
chapter 3. 'That experience started me thinking about leading life as
a single woman, and possibly having children on my own. I'd rather
live alone and have female friendships. And if I want to have children
I'd do it outside of marriage.' Pam's delight that she had not lost
the ability to have children has also been discussed before in chapter
3 and earlier in this chapter. Although she was faced with the
formidable prospect of raising three young children while in a
wheelchair, she felt great comfort in the fact that she could still have
another child. 'Oh you have lost sensation and movement, but you
have not lost the power and the ability [. . .] in your own mind
you are still capable of that most female function. I think that is
probably a very reassuring thing for a woman. I can remember
thinking that meant that I was not so different after all.' Notional
fertility is important, even if it is never acted upon (Greer 1984,
p. 47).

Children may enhance our lives in ways that go far beyond
compliance with social obligations, yet the pleasures of parenting
can no longer be assumed for the people in this study. Although
advances in reproductive technologies have brought the hope of
fatherhood to many previously infertile men, the success rates arc
still very low, and the demands of the program would deter all but
the strong-hearted. The fact that some of the men in this study are
contemplating these procedures, and that Anthony has been successful, is evidence of the continuing importance of fatherhood in our
society. Although the women have lost far less than most of the men
in terms of sexual performance and the ability to bear children, these
possibilities may amount to Pyrrhic victories since other elements of

conventional femininity may deny women the opportunity to act on this potential. Appearance, for example, may impede the development of an intimate relationship, the usual precursor of both sexual and reproductive activities. Even the women's fertility—the capacity for motherhood—may be subsumed in the face of assumptions about the women's diminished ability to nurture and care for others (Link 1987, pp. 26–7; Shaul et al. 1985)—the substance of motherhood. Children—having children, rearing children, worrying about children, not having children (Lewis 1986)—are critical issues.

The idea that motherhood is essential for, and desired by, all women (Rowland 1988, p. 166) is a compelling myth, but fathering a child is still a critical component of hegemonic masculinity (Connell 1983). Ideas of normality and abnormality are tied to the rigid parameters of the male–female dichotomy. Gendered sexuality demands that an individual must fit either a male or a female category; those people who do not fit must be abnormal, diseased or perverted (Kaplan & Rogers 1990, p. 225). As long as reproduction and sexuality remain tied to hegemonic masculinity, a body that is different will been seen as a problem for an individual to bear, rather than as an issue of central importance in the politics of the body. The presence and aliveness of the bodies of the people in this study confront such gendered categories.

6   Coping with embarrassment: bodily continence

'As far as one can tell there are no human societies where the act of excretion and its products are not subject to public and private arrangements, to expectations involving time and space, regularity and appropriateness' (Loudon 1977, p. 168). Routine bodily functions of micturition, defecation and menstruation seem cloaked in secrecy. Not only does the management of these activities take place behind closed doors, but beyond crude jokes or clinical situations, civilised behaviour provides few opportunities to openly discuss these topics. Talking about such things makes people feel uncomfortable; embarrassment, humiliation and shame compound the furtive, hidden nature of the activities. No one escapes the need to eliminate bodily wastes, yet these routine functions are often hidden in euphemism and furtive behaviour. Propriety has created disgust at the normal activities of healthy bodies.

THE BODY AND SOCIETY

The processes of civilisation depended on the management of bodily functions and bodily products. Beginning around the eleventh century, Elias traces the gradual incorporation of bodily functions into beliefs about acceptable 'civilised' behaviour (Elias 1978, p. 129). Concomitant with the 'civilising' of the body was the development of the concept of modesty, the acknowledgment of the need to privatise the 'private parts' of the body (Elias 1978, pp. 131–2). The sequestering of particular parts and functions of the body that are 'best not talked about' makes people vulnerable to embarrassment and shame should concealment fail (Elias 1978, p. 190). Despite Elias's sense of a linear civilising process, it is clear that particular presentations of a modest, 'civilised' body arise in all societies at different times, and that each society has a sense of the kind of bodily acts or parts of the body that threaten that particular civilisation (Douglas 1966, p. 121).

The anthropology of Mary Douglas has also been influential in establishing the relationship between the body and society. In *Purity and Danger* (1966) Douglas argues that the body provides a basic schema for political and moral symbolism. Ideas about pollution, defilement and transgression impose order on inherently untidy experience. 'It is only by exaggerating the difference between within and without, above and below, male and female, with and against, that a semblance of order is created' (Douglas 1966, p. 4). Parts and functions of the body associated with excretion and sex dominate this schema which, though culturally specific, is constant in the relationship it posits between concepts of pollution, the body and society.

Bodily orifices are especially worrisome (Douglas 1966, p. 121). Entrances and exits evoke danger because of their critical role in protecting society from intrusion by outsiders (Douglas 1973). In Douglas's work the body provides a metaphor of coherence and disorder. For this reason Turner claims that this work is not so much an anthropology of the body, as an anthropology of the symbolism of risk (Turner 1992, p. 51). In complex societies such as our own we seldom acknowledge the anxiety and rituals associated with bodily orifices—yet such places are heavily circumscribed with meaning and special practices. The concerns and practices cannot be explained in terms of individual psychology. We must be 'prepared to see in the body a symbol of society, and to see the powers and dangers credited to social structure reproduced in small on the human body' (Douglas 1966, p. 115). Although Douglas's work is most insightful, it threatens to reduce the phenomenology of the lived body into the positions and categories of the social body (Shilling 1993, p. 73).

Ideas of cleanliness, hygiene, purity and pollution relate to our sense of order and control. Dirt is, essentially, disorder. There is no such thing as absolute dirt. Dirt is relative to order. 'Dirt is a by-product of a systematic ordering and classification of matter in so far as ordering involves rejecting inappropriate elements' (Douglas 1966, p. 35). Shoes, for example, are not dirty in themselves but it is dirty to put them on the sofa. Vegetables are not dirty when growing in the garden, but become so when brought to the kitchen;

on a chair clothes are clean, on the floor they are dirty (Douglas 1966, p. 36). Matter out of place offends our sense of order. We are distressed by displaced matter.

It is not surprising that there is a close relationship between our ideas of cleanliness and purity and the excretory and sexual functions of the body. Our social anxieties reach their full height in relation to these bodily activities. The civilising forces of society constrain the body, yet these activities may subvert this control. Nursing is designated 'dirty work' because it involves direct contact with the body or body products (Lawler 1991, p. 47). Aversion to touching the normal products of well-functioning bodies—urine, faeces, saliva, blood, phlegm, nasal discharge, sweat—is part of childhood learning. A child is likely to be reprimanded for touching these 'dirty' body secretions. Similarly, a child exploring his or her bodily orifices may be told 'not to be dirty'. Bodily substances are, presumably, 'clean' in the body where they are produced, and 'clean' in the toilet, bedpan, urinal or handkerchief—their 'proper' destination. They become 'dirty' in transit from body to receptacle, and in their progress they dirty the orifice through which they pass to the outside world. Breasts, genitals, anus, armpits, nostrils, throat thus become 'dirty' by association. Small wonder that we grow up with a disgust of the normal healthy functioning of our bodies. To be taught to shun and hate the products of our own bodies is true alienation.

The vagina, the anus and the penis are especially vulnerable orifices. Matter issuing from these openings has the potential to provoke extreme anxiety. Blood, urine, faeces, semen and vaginal secretions, produced within the body, leave from these portals which mediate between the interior and exterior worlds of the body. Not surprisingly, intercourse, micturition, defecation and menstruation are bodily activities of great concern. Despite their intimate and private nature, such activities are highly regulated. Children are trained from an early age in strategies of body management (Turner 1987, p. 85); toilet training is a major task of child rearing. Enormous creative energy, and despair, go into the process. The parental elation accompanying baby's first dry night, and the joy at the sight of the first well-placed excrement, are testimony to the importance placed on bodily continence in our society. Once these lessons are learned and the potentially disruptive activities of the bowel and the bladder are subdued, the child can go on to attend to other, more mature activities.

A stable body relies on fixed sites of corporeal permeability and impermeability (Butler 1990, p. 132). Practices that redirect attention to particular areas of the body, or redefine the expectations of activities previously taken for granted, threaten to disrupt the stability of the body. Continence is, in effect, the conquest of the body by society. Society civilises the body to conform to its conventions. However, the truce between the body and society is always precarious. Bodily continence can never be taken for granted. Anxieties about continence reflect our perpetual fear that the body may defy its social conditioning and reassert its supremacy over our civilised learning. Faith in bodily processes, and particularly in the ability of the body's orifices to retain excremental matter until a socially convenient time and place is, at best, uneasy. Occasional attacks of diarrhoea are unsettling. Uncontrollable bowel activities strip adults of their civilised veneer and may render them as helpless as children. Urinary incontinence is an extremely common problem for women after the physical traumas of childbirth, and also for men as they grow older. Enormous industries thrive on the provision of disposable napkins to mop up infant excretions. These products are well advertised and promoted despite their disastrous effect on the environment. Yet the public nature of infant urinary and faecal management contrasts with the secrecy that shrouds adult incontinence, a much more disruptive and less temporary issue. The physical discomfort of a leaky bladder must be immense, but the stigma associated with the failure to guard one's bodily orifices is far greater. Shame and humiliation lead people to engage in elaborate strategies for concealment, including social withdrawal. Recurring anxieties about bodily continence stand in stark contrast to the limited opportunities society gives us to talk about such fears. Our bodies are held in perpetual and uneasy tension with society. Embarrassment is never far away.

THE IMPACT OF INCONTINENCE ON THE EMBODIED SELF

While the motor damage experienced by the people in this study is obvious, few people realise that bladder and bowel function are also involved. Even those people who know that these basic bodily functions can be implicated, think that these activities can be 'fixed up' in the rehabilitation period, that the problem can be solved. Yet such issues are recurring problems for these people throughout their lives, and many people claim that it is incontinence, particularly bladder incontinence, that is the most disruptive aspect of their condition (Morris 1989, ch. 10).

Most people with spinal cord damage no longer feel when their bladder needs emptying. The person must learn to interpret other 'feelings' that the bladder is full, and develop techniques to empty it. Bowel control is also lost. Bowel training, like the bowel training of childhood, aims to condition the bowel to produce regular

evacuations at the same time every day or every second day at a
time that is convenient to the person's lifestyle. But it is this necessity
for a life-long preoccupation with bodily eliminations that many of
the people in this study claim is the worst problem of all. Even those
men and women whose bladder and bowel functions are unimpaired
must still deal with the difficulties associated with lack of movement,
sensation or access. Having to rely on others to assist in these basic
bodily functions is an extremely damaging factor in the maintenance
of self-identity. The vulnerability of the paralysed person to the
vagaries affecting the lives of those people he or she must depend
on for care is a constant source of anxiety. Whether such people are
paid professional workers, friends, family, or lover, the obligations
engendered in this kind of intimate work may be enormous.

It is paradoxical that incontinence, the least talked about aspect
of the bodily damage, may have the most destructive impact on the
embodied self. As Anthony says:

> *It is one of the things least talked about—the bladder and bowels
> part of it. People talk about paras and quads, their lack of
> movement and their manual abilities, but what really impacts
> most is that area. The worst part of the disability is the loss of
> bodily function in those particular areas. If you can manage that,
> and control it well, it improves your quality of life so much.*

Bob agrees with Anthony that

> *the bladder and bowel problems predominate. If you took away
> the bladder and bowel problems it would be what some people
> think. Many families of newly disabled people think that it is
> just a matter of legs—so that all they have to do is lift the person
> from here to here and they will be all right.*

Although Frances's incontinence was a temporary condition in
the early part of her severe viral illness, she agrees that it was

> *terrible. They had to remove the catheter because of a urinary
> tract infection, and they said, 'Look, just wet the bed'. I had no
> control over it anyway, but I was mortified every time it hap-
> pened. I hated the fact that people had to come to change the
> sheets. It was just awful, and it was also so difficult for them to
> lift me because I could do nothing to help. It was an awful
> process. My bowels were horrific. I was being fed through a nasal
> gastric tube, and I hadn't had a bowel movement for weeks. I
> can remember that I was smelly, I was just vile, the gas that was
> coming from me was just terrible. So then I had enemas—series*

and series of enemas, those awful hand enemas. Even after I got out of intensive care they had to continue because I did not have bowel function for some time. It was an excruciating process. I remember saying, 'I'll have a baby anytime, anytime rather than go through this process'. I found the bowel enemas just vile.

Frances's loss of bowel and bladder control was, mercifully, temporary. After the initial acute phase of the illness had passed, these functions returned. Most of the men and women, however, have not been so lucky. For George, too, the loss of bladder and bowel function has been 'the biggest thing you have to come to terms with. In my particular case it has taken until now, and a major operation to sort my bladder out. It has taken three years of determined effort to convince medical people what I want.' Ken is particularly angry with the way the doctors dealt with his bowel retraining when he first damaged his body some seven years ago. As Ken says:

The single biggest difficulty I had was the whole issue of bowel and bladder control and the management of those functions. Because I am a paraplegic, they felt that I might be able to get my bladder working again through straining or whatever. That just did not work. Coupled with that was my difficulty with bowel control. I don't know if it is different anywhere else, but all doctors seem to have this obsession with keeping bowels open, and I believe that they have this obsession at the expense of your normal functioning in society. One of the most demeaning and belittling things is not having control over your bowels. It creates enormous feelings of powerlessness. And yet while I was there [in the rehabilitation unit], *I was having accidents daily—more than daily—and it was associated with physical movement. I was going through rehabilitation—lifting weights, trying to stand up, walking between parallel bars and stuff like that. Every time I did anything physical, my bowels would move—not much some-times, but enough to create a helluva mess and a smell. So I would have to find a nurse to clean me up and I'd have to get changed. I was running out of clothes. And all the time they are giving me coloxyl with danthron, and they are also giving me suppositories every other morning. Now here we are seven years down the track—and it hasn't taken that long to resolve it—but seven years down the track and I don't take anything. I don't use suppositories, and I don't take metamucil or any kind of fibre-bulk things. I don't take any kind of medication that is associated with bowel care whatever.*

Mary, too, claims that issues associated with disrupted bowel and bladder function and control are the most significant aspects of her bodily loss. She remembers saying to her father in the very early days of her rehabilitation, I'll never walk to the toilet. In exasperation, her father said, '"Look, why on earth do you have to reduce everything to toilet level?". Well you do. That's life if your bowels and bladder are involved. If those areas are sorted out then life's a breeze.'

Despite the lack of knowledge and general understanding about these issues, the impact of the loss of these basic functions is profound. The changed function not only causes a host of difficult practical problems, but more significantly, it is a fundamental challenge to embodiment and to the manner in which the person is able to reconstitute his or her embodied self. It may be that it is our own fears of bodily incontinence that prevent us from seeing these losses as anything more than practical issues of bodily input and output: as technical problems of bodily plumbing that, with a bit of patience and self-regulation, can be resolved. While dreadful to think about, most of us can begin to imagine what it may be like not to be able to move our legs. To confront the spectre of incontinence may be too terrible to contemplate.

Anthony considers himself very fortunate because he has some sensory sparing which means that 'I know when I need to go to the toilet, so I don't need to have that form of bladder and bowel management. I know people who have had to have that all these years. I would have found that extremely difficult—the inconvenience and the time.' Anthony goes on to say: 'I know the great joy and excitement I had when I started to be able to go to the toilet and use my bowels again—the sensation and the feeling!' Anthony's elation at achieving what seem such mundane goals after two years of effort highlights the dramatic impact of this aspect of bodily damage.

When discussing the impact of his loss of bladder and bowel function with me, Alister's phrase that it was 'a bit of a pain in the arse at times', while colourful in expression, was in fact extremely imprecise in description. It is because of the lack of sensation of all kinds 'in the arse' that this loss is so difficult to manage. The meaning, however, was quite clear:

> It is similar to being a child. It may have taken you eighteen months to learn bladder and bowel control as a child. Perhaps being an adult gives you the opportunity of learning a little bit quicker, but that's about all. You've got to start training your bowel and bladder all over again using the different methods people use, and you have got to work out an option that suits yourself the best.

Bridget is unequivocal that the loss of bladder and bowel function was the worst aspect of her disability, although this is becoming less distressing for her as time passes: 'I felt pretty bad about that. It was a real challenge to get the catheter in the right place at first. I used to have a lot of misses. I had to wear these big nappies at first. Bowel care is really difficult. With the suppositories you flood all over the toilet. It was a real hassle.' George feels that the worst impact of bowel and bladder loss is the 'abnormality of it all'. The difficulties associated with having to ask other people to help him in these basic activities took its toll on George. For several years he 'didn't go anywhere because it was just too hard'. Now he can manage all the aspects of bowel and bladder function himself: 'Now I feel more normal. If I go to a venue with my mates, it saves a lot of explanation if I can take care of all of these things myself.' Joy, too, feels this loss most profoundly. She says: 'I miss the feeling of wanting to go to the toilet, you know, you miss things like that—the feeling of a full bladder or just going to the toilet. I dream about it all the time. In my dreams it's so real, it feels like it's real.'

Mark still remembers the harsh, early problems of bowel and bladder loss:

> I remember the pain associated with the change from having an in-dwelling catheter to using condom drainage. I remember once I was up in Belair National Park with friends when the catheter got blocked. I had to get them to race me back to the hospital to have the catheter changed. Then there was the mess, you know, shitting myself—having accidents—and that went on for quite a number of years after I left the unit.

MANAGING BODILY INCONTINENCE

The practical management of incontinence is a never-ending problem.

Bridget now wears pads for the urinary incontinence and uses suppositories from time to time to assist in the evacuation of her bowel. She can feel her bladder, as she says:

> My bladder is what they call a spastic bladder. It has spasms by itself. After I have a drink I can feel it filling up. Even when I feel it is full, it can take another twenty mils. It doesn't take as much as it used to, it has shrunk. Because I get spasms all the time, it creates a muscular wall, and as this muscular wall gets bigger the inside gets smaller, and therefore it can't hold as much urine.

George has a similar type of bladder condition to Bridget. He has recently had an operation to remedy some aspects of this. In his words:

> I had a bladder augmentation operation, which consists of removing a segment of bowel and cutting the bladder open and stitching it into the bladder. That changes the characteristics of your bladder from being a spastic bladder which meant that it didn't have a very big volume and it was prone to uncontrolled contractions which meant that you voided uncontrollably. This operation fixes the tone of the bladder and also enlarges the capacity which, to put it mildly, has been a marvellous change. But it took up to now to convince the powers that be that this is what I needed.

As Mary says:

> The problems associated with bowel and bladder are endless. I have just wet myself now talking to you—not because I have been talking to you, but because I have had a cup of coffee. I would love to wear pretty underwear, but what I must wear are babies' nappies. I didn't give away Ann's nappies, and when my sister-in-law's children grew out of nappies she passed them on to me.

It wasn't until Pam returned home after nine months in the rehabilitation unit that she was able to work out ways of managing her wayward bladder to fit with her own lifestyle:

> When I came home I said to Phillip, 'Now we have to go through this process of measuring what I drink'. I used to sit on the portable commode by the hour just finding out how long it took to come through and then measure it. We did all this testing ourselves for months until I learned control. Now I can lead a very flexible life. Of course I can still have accidents. I might not be able to have access to a toilet when I need it, or I might be lazy and not get there when I should. I might drink more than is wise because I am socialising, but I try to be very careful, and my bladder is fairly reliable. You have to make allowances for winter and summer, and from time to time you may not be well, but over the years I've learned all that. It was about six months after I returned home that I began to develop some confidence in my bladder.

Bob has not had control of his bowels since his accident.

I cannot feel that I need to go to the toilet, nor can I go by myself. You get taught a routine though, that has really worked well for me. When I first went home I found that if I drank too much beer I was in all sorts of trouble with diarrhoea. Gradually I learned to control this—I got to know my body. What I do now is that I know that I have to go every two days. I have learned this technique of tightening my stomach muscles and I go—which is very lucky. I hear of other people who have to have suppositories then sit over a toilet for ages. That seems like the most boring thing I could think of, whereas it takes me about the same time that it would take a normal person. Although I have some problems from time to time, I think that I am very lucky in that way.

Although Ken doesn't use any kind of medication associated with bowel care now, he still remembers the anguish his bowel retraining caused him:

The issue for me is that they knew what the medications they had prescribed for me were doing. They knew the difficulties that I was having every day and the embarrassment that it caused me, and yet their obsession with keeping my bowels open and moving was such that they disregarded all that and kept me on the medication and never explained to me what that medication was doing. If I had known then what I know now about the action of the different medication they were using I would have been more assertive. I guess that there are a lot of people who would say, 'How could he have been more assertive or more aggressive than he was when he was in hospital anyway?' because I was already deemed to be pretty obnoxious. But if I had been more assertive about that process I'd have found out exactly what it did do and I would have told them to 'stick it' and I wouldn't have taken the medication any more and got things under control a whole lot earlier.

It took Ken at least another year after he had left the rehabilitation unit to 'get it sorted out to my satisfaction. For the first six months when I went home I was wearing a "bluey" stuffed down inside my jocks, changing it sometimes several times a day because I was having continual bowel accidents. And all this time I was taking coloxyl.' A 'bluey', Ken explains,

is a hospital pad with blue plastic liner and absorbent material on the other side. You are not supposed to wear anything like that next to your skin if you are a paraplegic because of the

*potential for pressure sore problems or skin irritations. But it
was the only way that I could function. And even then I was
changing these things a minimum of once a day, sometimes twice,
three, four times or more. Ultimately I chucked all this stuff
away. Now I have bowel accidents infrequently, unless I am sick.
It is nowhere near the problem it was. I am still really angry
about that and the way the doctors dealt with that.*

Although Mary claims that bladder problems are endless she
continues, more forcefully, to say:

*but I don't think that there is a word bad enough to describe
the problems associated with the bowel. Swear words don't even
cover the vicious feelings I have. If there were anything more
vicious than swear words I'd use them. Bladder training is a
euphemism. It doesn't train your bladder at all—it just means
that you beat your bladder to it. As far as my bowels are
concerned, I go once a day. Something may or may not happen,
and it's a revolting process. I've been down the suppository track.
I have ended up having to do it with a gloved hand—what's
called 'manual removal'. In my case it's a very messy occupation,
and it prevents me going away to stay overnight. What on earth
would I do if I found myself with a toilet that is unsuitable, and
I made an awful mess that I'd have to clean up? It is all right,
because my own bathroom is equipped for it. My biggest fear is
that someone else will have to be involved in all of this. Diarrhoea, let me tell you, is no fun. It's awful, and it's terribly
distressing.*

Rosemary has an ileostomy bag for urinary elimination; faecal
material, though, must be manually removed from her bowel. Her
mother has done this for her all her life, but as Rosemary says, 'Now
I am getting older I should try to do this for myself'. Rosemary has
been able to develop a very predictable routine in this regard: 'I have
manual removal twice a week at nights, and it generally takes about
half an hour to empty my bowels'. Unlike many of the people in
this study, Rosemary is seldom distressed by the practical issues
associated with her lack of bladder and bowel function: 'The only
problem I have as far as the bladder goes is if the urine bag comes
off, or it leaks. But I can just change it while I am on my bed with
a mirror and stuff.' Her overwhelming desire to appear as much like
her friends as possible, though, means that Rosemary actively avoids
discussion of bodily eliminations with others.
    An incomplete lesion, coupled with a successful program of
bladder and bowel retraining, enabled Sally to manage her own

bladder and bowel by the time she left the unit. She can feel when she needs to urinate or pass a bowel motion, so she is able to press on her stomach to assist evacuation. Although she does not require mechanical assistance at the moment, she anticipates that she may need to explore other methods to facilitate these processes as she becomes older, or if she has a child.

Unlike many people in the study, Alister claims that he was not distressed by the rigorous, formal program of bladder and bowel management that is central to spinal injury rehabilitation. He was able to see the catheterisation and suppositories 'as practical measures which just had to be done. Well you have no choice. You either do it or you don't cope.' Alister's phlegmatic attitude towards this aspect of rehabilitation is rare; most of the men and women perceive the implications and practices arising from this loss as a destructive incursion into their embodied selves, and a recurring attack on their bodily integrity and self-esteem throughout their lives. Jenny talks about the indignities of adult incontinence. Her experiences are similar to those of Frances, discussed earlier. Jenny says:

> With the lack of bladder control, you were constantly having to have your sheets changed—every few hours, day and night. I found all of that a real intrusion. There were lots and lots of jokes—'Oh you're wet again', and 'Didn't your mother toilet train you?', or whatever. And I remember one nurse really swearing and saying, 'Oh bloody women, you can never find their urethra'. I can remember being very disturbed about this issue of the difficulty that some of the staff had about inserting a catheter into the female anatomy. I was very distressed about the level of intrusion, and also at the level of patient blaming.

Anthony, too, describes his distress at the level of dependence on the staff incurred by his loss of control of bodily evacuation and continence:

> Every second night you would have to go down to have 'bombs' [suppositories]. After that there was no negotiation about staying up, you would have to go straight to bed. You were sitting on the toilet for an age, but the orderlies would never agree to dress you again. If you wanted to stay up you had to stay up with just a shirt or a jumper on and a sheet wrapped around you. It was very uncomfortable, so most people went to bed.

Infections can be a perpetual problem for people with disordered urinary function. As Bob says, 'I have been getting lots of bladder infections in the last three years, and it is mainly a drainage problem'.

He has recently had a supra-pubic catheter put in: 'This means that you have a pipe coming out of your stomach. It takes a bit of getting used to, but it means that your penis is free, and more importantly, you are less likely to get infections.' Some time before this procedure Bob had what is called a bladder nick. This, however, did not solve the problem and, in fact, it created another problem. 'They nick the sphincter and the bladder to make the flow better, but when they did this to me I lost part of my erection. I thought, "They won't do that again to me!".'

Anthony says that it was many years before he felt comfortable with his body again: 'One of the things that really affected my sexuality was that for about the first seven years I wore a condom and an external drainage bag. I found that really affected me—my body and my sexuality—I found that really difficult. I now use intermittent catheterisation and water flow management, so I don't need anything extra.' Bob, too, found great difficulty in reconciling the external plumbing apparatus with his embodied self. Bob discussed his difficulties in maintaining an existing relationship during his time in the rehabilitation unit in an earlier chapter. A major component of this difficulty was

> *my thoughts about how my lady would respond to a piece of tube hanging off the end of my penis, and my own feelings about it as well. I remember that we tried a few times taking the condom drainage off. But she got a couple of bladder infections from it, so that discouraged her, and understandably me as well. It was very hard to have a normal relationship under such conditions. I think that is why so many people go to self-catheterisation now. You don't have to wear anything except when you do the catheter, and you are free from urinating when you don't want to.*

Although Ken's experiences with his bowels were particularly difficult, he fared better when it came to bladder management. In common with most people with paraplegia, Ken has the full range of movement and power in his upper limbs. His finger dexterity enables him to use self-catheterisation techniques: 'I have been very happy with that. I do four catheters a day, which is roughly one every six hours. Now I don't have chronic urinary tract infections and if I do get an infection then I drink more and I do more catheters.'

Gendered experience of bodily incontinence

The practical problems associated with disrupted bodily continence are complicated and never-ending, the impact on embodiment is immense. Does the particular anatomical structure of male or female genital and urinary organs influence the experience of this loss? Is this bodily disorder experienced differently for men and women in terms of conventional gender categories? The technical accoutrements of bowel and bladder management alone may vary the impact of this loss for a man or a woman. It is still overwhelmingly women's role to assume primary responsibility for the housekeeping of the 'body' of the family—for managing the effluvia, dirt and waste in the family (Martin 1987, p. 201). While this responsibility may increase a woman's familiarity with such issues, it may also exacerbate the difficulties women may have in accommodating the disorder and chaos in their own bodies.

A critical task associated with child rearing is the responsibility for the training of children in bodily continence. A dry napkin and a properly placed bowel action are major milestones. Such achievements are indicators of substantial childhood maturity; a position that can now be taken for granted, and from which one never expects to retreat. Yet, in the situation of bodily disruption, the teacher and manager of others is herself out of control. To find oneself, as an adult, again in the world of baby napkins, dirty bed linen, soiled clothing, unpleasant odours, and having to attend to eating and drinking regimes, skin irritations and the whereabouts of the toilet, is a grave assault on a woman's self-esteem. To have to constantly attend to these things that are associated with the very early stages of child rearing and with very small babies is extremely destructive to the embodied self. Painstaking though infant bladder and bowel training may seem, it is a relatively predictable procedure, undertaken with the clear expectation that continence is possible, and that the hard work of discipline and regimes of food and liquid intake will be rewarded. In a relatively short time the child will be trained. Adult training comes with no such assurances. At times it may seem that some degree of control has been achieved, only for it to be lost at a later stage. Infections, and other associated issues, continually confound the best efforts at management.

A woman's conventional associations with the bowel and bladder training of others may make the impact of her own incontinence worse, but do men fare any better in respect to disordered bodily continence? Masculinity is also a formidable construction. It may be this same issue that makes loss of bowel and bladder function also hard for a man to bear. Men's traditional dissociation from these tasks of managing bodily continence usually assumed by women may be the issue that makes men's loss so difficult to bear. Changing dirty napkins gives no one pleasure, yet women still most often accommodate this task as one of the obligations of parenthood. The world of soiled clothing and wet bed linen is not a world with which men are normally familiar. To be suddenly plunged into a world with which you never expected to be involved, and from which you were protected in infancy by the ministrations of your own mother, is a rude and bitter shock for many men.

As if gender roles were not enough, phallocentrism presents another serious blow for men in this area of intimate activities. Under this construction, a man's penis is the source of his masculine strength and identity. A strong stream of urine has been part of men's mythology since infant school days. In *Love in the Time of Cholera*, for example, Márquez describes the reaction of Fermina Daza to the sound of her husband's urination on their wedding night. She thinks 'The sound of his stallion's stream seemed so potent, so replete with authority'. As he becomes older, Dr Urbino reminisces that 'his stream was so defined and so direct that when he was at school he won contests for marksmanship in filling bottles'. As his stream became 'oblique and scattered' he would say 'The toilet must have been invented by someone who knew nothing about men'. As an old man the solution was for him to urinate sitting down, as his wife did, 'which kept the bowl clean and him in a state of grace' (Márquez 1988, p. 30).

Being able to hit the back of the lavatory wall at ten paces brings instant fame to boys in the schoolyard. The embarrassment many older men feel at having to front up to an open urinal is part of this same need to display a large penis and a strong stream of urine. The conflation of the size of the penis and the strength of the flow of urine with sexual prowess is illogical, yet persistent. To defile this organ which is the site of so many meanings with the trappings of bladder management is a very real tragedy for most men. To come to feel so unhappy about this part of the body with which men are supposed to feel so pleased is a significant part of the losses that men must feel.

Although he has suffered a lot himself, Anthony sympathises with women in relation to these issues: 'It seems much more difficult for them, even if they have the ability to self-catheterise, it is a much more difficult procedure for women than for males. If they have to have an in-dwelling catheter, it must have quite a profound effect on them, I am sure.' Like Anthony, George agrees that these things would be much harder for a woman, 'especially with all the associated female problems that they have to deal with'. Peter, too, agrees that 'it is a lot more difficult for a woman. A woman has to deal with the constant odour, I suppose, and things like that males don't have trouble with.'

How do the women perceive their own problems in comparison with the problems experienced by men?

Jenny says: 'Men might have difficulty with female nurses attaching things to their penises and so on (an issue discussed in Lawler 1991, pp. 199–202), but for me the issue of constant incontinence was the most difficult thing to bear'. The difficulties experienced by staff in finding a woman's urethra, an issue already discussed, presented another disadvantage not experienced by men. Joy says: 'Well, a man has to insert a catheter a lot further than a woman does. On the other hand if a man is wearing a leg bag he can just go into a dark corner and empty it out. It would be a bit embarrassing for a woman to do this if she wore a catheter.' Mary feels 'that it is much harder for women than for men because men have something convenient to attach something to. I've now gone on to intermittent catheters, which makes it quicker in many ways. A lot of men can do that too.' Mary goes on to say:

> The bowel side of things would be similar for a man and a woman, but in general men are better off. In part it is because they don't have menstruation attached. But mainly it is because they have got something that is easier to get at, that they can do themselves, even if they are quadriplegic men. Women have to get on to something to pass urine. You really have to undress to get at what is underneath—and that in itself can be a real hassle. If the fly is big enough in men's clothing, they can get at it.

Fungal vaginal infection can be a difficult issue for all women. The likelihood of such infections is much greater for women with disturbances such as these, and the techniques involved in management of the infection exacerbate the problem. Mary says: 'You have to get into bed to put all the various suppositories and creams in, then you have to get up afterwards to go and clean up. It is not easy to put these things in, and it is not easy to clean up afterwards then get back into bed without losing it all. You can't feel or see what you are doing—you have to do it with mirrors.'

Beyond these seemingly relentless practical problems though, Mary raises an issue that may be central to women's difficulties in this area. She says:

> When I was in hospital for so long, I remember a quadriplegic lady who, because of her disability, was very dependent. I remember her first few weekends at home when she first had to get her husband to do these things. He had to sort out her menstruation and sort out her catheters—but she was even more mortified when he had to put his gloved hand into her rectum to sort out her bowel problems. Suppositories or no suppositories, he still had to do it, and she was mortified by this. She used to come back from weekends, distressed beyond measure. She said

to me after one such occasion, 'I can't even kill myself—I am physically unable to kill myself'. She is now, a dozen years later, a very well-adjusted lady, with a very happy relationship with her husband who is still with her.

Conventional roles for women are so closely associated with caring for a male partner that a reversal of this situation—a man having to take care of a woman, especially in relation to intimate care—is intolerable for many women. Personal care could become a significant aspect of re-embodiment, although none of the informants in this study claimed that it had been so for them. In the literature, several women with severe disabilities claim that the fact that their sexual partner is also responsible for their personal care 'is a very deep and strong part of our relationship, part of our loving, and part of our sexuality and sensuality. It's just a very natural part of what our relationship is' (Fishwick 1981, p. 121).

Although many men assume major responsibility for the care of sick or ageing women and for children, such expectations are still not the usual expectations men have of their lives in Western society at the end of the twentieth century (Braithwaite 1990). For a man to confront the unusual possibility that he may have to be the life-long carer of a woman may be an extremely difficult aspect of rehabilitation. The difficulties women face in allowing this to happen may also be a major impediment to their own re-embodiment. The necessity of depending on others to manage those parts and functions of the body seen as private and intimate, even from one's own partner, is a most severe attack on bodily integrity and self-esteem. Feelings of passion and pleasure usually associated with the genital area become confused by the sense of shame and embarrassment at having to involve a partner in such basic activities. To maintain a sense of self in the face of such constant incursions requires exceptional personal skills and self-knowledge, rare in most of us, and by no means a prerequisite for the onset of serious bodily disorder.

Menstrual blood has always been associated with danger and risk. Emanating from 'the wicked womb' (Greer 1970, p. 47), hidden in the dark interior of a woman's body and discharged from the body through the dangerous vaginal orifice, no other bodily substance has been invested with such symbolism or so many social prohibitions. Obviously, menstruation is a bodily function that presents men and women with different experiences in the task of remaking their bodies. Frances speaks of the irony that her menstrual period continued despite the massive disruption that was occurring to her body. She says:

Within days of going into intensive care I menstruated. I can remember being furious, and thinking, 'My God, my body is failing me in every way, surely this way can fail too!'. By the time I got to the rehabilitation stage my periods had settled in very strong and fast again. Not being able to change your own pads and things like that was horrific. I needed help being lifted on and off the lavatory, obviously, and I had to have a male nurse to do it because my body was so floppy. Some people would come in and just put their arms around me and think that they could hold me, but I would slip through people's arms. I would end up on the floor, and they would wonder where I had gone. So I always had this male nurse, who was very good, to take me to the lavatory, but I found dealing with the menstruation thing horrific.

Mary, too, talks of the problems associated with the recurring cycles of menstruation. She says:

As if the problems associated with bladder and bowels are not enough, you have to cope with the extra tasks involved in menstruation. In fact I have recently had a hysterectomy because I had fibroids and my periods were getting heavier, more frequent and irregular. I wasn't really at the stage of desperately needing a hysterectomy, but I said to the gynaecologist, 'Is there any point in going on? I am going to end up needing one. Please do it now'. The relief is absolutely wonderful—it has solved one of the recurring dilemmas.

Pam was 'as regular as anything with my periods' and didn't find the management of this bodily activity particularly difficult because 'I wear a sanitary pad all the time anyway in case of accidents'. Rosemary, too, does not find managing menstrual blood particularly difficult: 'I do get pretty heavy periods, and I would rather not have them, but I can change my own pads. I can kneel on the floor and change them myself.'

Tina has experienced the gradual deterioration of her body since childhood. It is interesting to note that when asked to comment on the issue of menstruation Tina chose not to discuss practical issues of menstrual management as the other women had done, but to suggest that for her, menstruation is an important confirmation of womanhood. She says:

Menstruation is a funny thing because I got very mixed messages as a child. When I first menstruated, all the teachers at school were saying, 'You're a woman now, Tina—it's great! it's lovely!'. And when I went home my mother said, 'Don't tell anybody you've got it, especially don't tell the boys'. So I got very mixed messages. I was pretty much caught between two societies. Consequently, I thought menstruation was a bad thing. So I went on the Pill when I was twenty-one so that I didn't have to have it. I didn't have to put up with those awful things. About eighteen months ago [about ten years later] I went off the Pill. I thought, I don't really want to go back on that. I am quite happy to have my periods now.

The practical tasks of managing menstruation are immense for women such as Tina, yet it is clear that for some women this central affirmation of bodiliness transcends the many difficulties that may be involved. The importance attributed to menstruation by Tina is substantiated by other women with severe bodily disruption in a recent survey (ACROD, 1988).

IMPACT OF BODILY INCONTINENCE ON RELATIONSHIPS

Body boundaries are dangerous; body orifices are particularly vulnerable (Douglas 1966). Bodily openings are concentrated in the perineum, a relatively small area of men's and women's bodies. Bodily secretions—semen, vaginal secretions, faeces, urine and blood—pass from the body through these exterior portals. These orifices also offer a pathway into the body for bacteriological, physical and moral invaders. Encumbered with the duty of protecting the body from infection, physical abuse and immorality, it is surprising that the genital area can also be a site of pleasure. The perils associated with bodily boundaries and orifices, with purity and defilement, with emotions and sensations are concentrated in this area. The role of body smells and body substances in the establishment and expression of significant relationships is well established (Loudon 1977, p. 169). Tensions created by genital organs, already heavily endowed with sensory receptors, are enhanced by the bodily secretions, sights and smells with which this place abounds.

For the most part, our lives are characterised by caution, restraint, prudence and sensible choices. Sexual activities may offer the opportunity to temporarily transcend the careful pragmatism of our daily lives, to escape the routines and responsibilities upon which social life depends and to smell the dangers and taste the pleasures of irresponsibility. Consorting with danger introduces us to the thrill of risk and vulnerability. The proximity to disease, the volatility of passion, and the potential for moral disorder may contribute to the excitement of sexual activities. It may be that it is 'the hint of catastrophe which makes sex bearable in the age of the death of seduction' (Kroker & Kroker 1988, p. 14). Teasing the senses, flirting with danger creates the *frisson* upon which sexual excitement depends.

While few able-bodied men and women are unaware of the volatile nature of the perineal area, most people develop a range of strategies to divert themselves and the attentions of others from this dangerous part of the body. People allow others to know only as much about the 'private parts' of their bodies as they feel comfortable to deal with. The disruption caused by unpredictable bowel and bladder actions cannot be ignored. The relentless concentration of energy and attention to the genital areas of the men and women in this study must surely interfere with other, more pleasurable activities associated with this area. How do these people reconcile their lifetime preoccupation with the management of bodily eliminations with their sexuality? Can new pleasures and sexualities arise in this context of risk, danger and uncertainty?

Anthony says:

> *Probably the main impediment to sexual performance and sexual activity is that you can't control when you urinate, nor do you know when you are using your bowels. It is very scary, and very threatening. The need to protect yourself means that you don't open up to people. Also there is that dissociation of parts of your body with particular activities. I found that it really affected me. I was certainly not comfortable with that. I found it really hard to reconcile my body with my sexuality.*

Bob has already discussed the impediments involved in 'thinking about how my lady would respond to a piece of tube hanging off my penis, and my own feelings about it as well'. The insertion of a supra-pubic catheter nearly a dozen years later (discussed earlier in this chapter) has relieved this situation. As Bob says: 'It takes a bit of getting used to, but it means that your penis is free'. Although George's accident was several years ago now, he claims that 'my main worries about approaching someone in order to develop a relationship are about my bowel and bladder. I am still sorting those things out. As you progress, you get more confident. Once you are in control of everything yourself, things change.'

Jenny speaks of her apprehension about recommencing a sexual relationship after her accident:

> *Oh, I was terrified, particularly about the incontinence problems. I remember I talked with one lady about how I would manage it, you know, the techniques of taking off the incontinence pad, and the stuff like the incontinence-type underwear. It would have*

*to be planned like, 'Shall we go to bed?' and 'I'll meet you in
the bed' so to speak. So I worked out that I'd go to the toilet
and take off this underwear last thing before jumping into bed.
So there I would be in bed without my knickers on, hoping like
hell that my bladder would not do something.*

Jenny's colourful description, though, does not disguise the disruptive effects of these early sexual encounters on embodiment.
Talking about the early days of her rehabilitation, Joy says:

*They train you in hospital. They lay you on a bed and give you
suppositories for bowel care. It's terrible, you lose all your
modesty—you know, shitting and urinating in front of people
and stuff like that. It really hurts your pride. Now, at night-time,
if Tom stays, I get embarrassed about this. I take a urine bottle
to bed and just lie in bed and catheterise myself. I get really
embarrassed about it, but it doesn't bother him. It doesn't bother
some guys, some guys wouldn't tell you if it did. That's a part
they have to accept about seeing me.*

Family attitudes and practices associated with nakedness, body
exposure and acceptable topics of conversation about the body are
governed by a range of socio-cultural variables (Lawler 1991,
p. 117). While nurses and many other health professionals may feel
awkward when performing certain tasks of bodily management for
others, it is often within the family that embarrassment about nudity
is felt most strongly. Most of the informants in Lawler's study
described a style of family life and upbringing where bodily functions
were dealt with in a 'civilised manner': sensitive bodily functions
were carried out in private, they were not discussed, and the body
was almost always kept covered (Lawler 1991, p. 118). Relationships
between parents and children are governed by complex informal rules
and expectations. Few families feel comfortable with nudity, yet
informal exposure of the body to casual acquaintances in the change
room, dressmaking class, or sauna may cause much less concern.
The spectre of one's parents wishing to 'speak to you about sex' is
one of the horrors of childhood. Intimate sexual detail, or the
minutiae of excretory function are seldom the subject of discussion
between family members after the brief years of infancy. Nudity in
the context of the family is more likely to provoke embarrassment
than complacency. How does the concept of self survive the necessity
of relying on one's children or parents to perform the intimate tasks
that are essential for survival?

Pressure areas and abscesses have been recurring problems for
Mary, as they are for many people with bodily paralysis. The last

time that she was in hospital she was able to come home earlier than usual because her children were now old enough to look after her. Mary discussed in chapter 3 how her son, Alan, helped her two daughters to lift me, soaking wet and stark naked, from under the shower onto my chair and how her daughters helped her to manage the tasks of catheterisation and dealing with menstruation. As Mary says, 'you can't have any secrets from your children'.

The impact of dependency on relationships has been discussed in chapter 3. Dependency is a continuous tension throughout the lives of people with damaged bodies, but the tension is heightened by the perpetual need to rely on others to carry out the intimate tasks of bodily maintenance necessary for survival. People with less extensive bodily damage have been able to become almost independent, but few escape the need to ask others for help, at least sometimes. Exchanging favours, helping each other out, sharing the tasks of everyday life is part of the fabric of social life. Seldom, though, are such acts the product of pure altruism. Underlying these transactions is a sense of reciprocity: the expectation that if I do this for you now, you will repay me, some time, in similar measure. The impossibility of being able to 'repay' a person for doing the tasks upon which one's life depends puts great strain on relationships.

When helping professionals help their patients, the nature of the help is determined by the professional person's interpretation of what the patient needs based on a professional model of treatment and management of such conditions. The reward for the professional worker is for the patient to get better, to manage for himself or herself; such goals fulfil professional ideals of success. The introduction of attendant care schemes in recent years has recognised the client's right to decide what needs to be done, to hire and fire the attendant, and to assume sole responsibility for the interaction (Lonsdale 1990, pp. 165–7). This model of care attempts to address many of the issues associated with dependency relationships. Yet the necessity of having the basic tasks of bodily survival executed by another person invests these issues with enormous risk and danger. Severely injured in mid-life, a male doctor compares the 'safety fears' he experienced 'in bed, in a wheelchair and on crutches' with the 'fears that many women must feel [. . .] of violence [. . .] of dependence [. . .] and of psychological depletion which any incessant fear can cause'. 'Injured men', he claims, 'begin to understand' (Moore 1991, p. 116). The potential for domestic abuse, harassment and emotional blackmail in situations where one person must depend on the ministrations of another is an additional burden for some people to bear (Breckenridge & Carmody 1992; Lonsdale 1990, pp. 6, 72).

Bodily continence is a critical component of embodiment. The

interrelationship between sexuality and continence has been dramatically highlighted by the experiences of the men and women in this
study. Mark still remembers 'the mess, the shitting myself, the
accidents that went on for quite a number of years after I had left
the unit'. Jenny's memories of the constantly wet bed in the early
stages of her rehabilitation are still vivid. Joy remembers the indignity
of 'shitting and urinating in front of people during bowel and bladder
retraining' as her worst humiliation. Ken's mortification at his bowel
accidents was profound: 'One of the most demeaning and belittling
things is not having control over your bowels. It creates a feeling of
complete powerlessness.' Ken is still angry with the way his doctors
dealt with this aspect of his rehabilitation. Rosemary tries very hard
to avoid any discussion of her bowel or bladder arrangements with
her friends: 'It is just too difficult for able-bodied people to cope
with'. Frances, too, was humiliated by her inability to control her
bladder and bowel: 'I was mortified every time I wet the bed. My
bowels were horrific. I hadn't had a bowel movement forever, and
I can remember that I was smelling vile—the gas that was coming
from me was just vile.'

The men and women will never forget the indignity and humiliation of these early events; these experiences cannot simply be
relegated to the past. Resolution of these disruptive issues is always
tentative: bladder and bowel routines must be obsessively main-
tained, equipment must be hygienically cleaned and stored, practices
and activities must be cautiously pursued. Infections, ageing, care-
lessness or haste can disrupt the fragile truce that these men and
women are able to strike with their anarchic bodily organs, and no
matter how hard they may try, some people may never achieve even
this most delicate détente.

Sexuality involves vulnerability, uncertainty and insecurity. We
live in fear that our bodies will let us down. We invest great trust
in our bodily orifices. Incontinence may be our worst nightmare.
The continual threat of danger and fear of bodily betrayal experienced by people in this study challenge the embodied self and impede
the on-going project of re-embodiment. To be constantly reminded
about those parts and functions of the body that most people try so
hard to forget is the burden that these people must bear. That many
of the people in this study have explored new sexualities and
developed novel erotic possibilities despite these disruptive activities
is testimony to their strength and resilience. Yet embarrassment,
shame, indignity and mortification are seldom far away.

7   A new body in a new world

This study has been an amazing journey. While often poignant, the informants' stories of intimate dimensions of their lives have revealed rich insights into human embodiment and the capacity of the body to survive crisis and disruption. Although seldom examined in everyday life, the aspects of embodiment that their experiences have exposed concern us all.

EMBODIMENT: UNDERSTANDING THE BODY IN SOCIETY

Body work is the principal activity of everyday life, and as embodied actors, we actively employ our bodies to create or alter the experience of being a body within a social world. Having and being a body lie at the core of all self-creation and world-building activities. As we participate in the continual task of re-embodiment throughout our lives we are, in effect, engaging in everyday rehabilitation. However, Scarry reminds us of the difficulties in comprehending the 'atrocities one's own body, muscle, and bone structure can inflict on oneself' (1985, p. 48), and Shilling writes, 'It is only in the context of the body's inevitable death that we can understand its full social importance' (1993, p. 175). The severe bodily damage experienced by the informants in this study highlights the taken-for-granted activities and experiences in which all bodies engage. These people's achievements celebrate the dynamic and integrative nature of embodiment.

The bodies in this study may seem weak and frail. In terms of the dominant construction of the biomedical body they are indeed sick, unhealthy, imperfect and abnormal bodies. Few of the bodies conform to conventional social categories relating to appearance, mobility, intimacy, sexuality, physicality or continence. Within the medicalised context of formal rehabilitation, such damage is viewed as a state of bodily imperfection, as a tragedy which the individual must accept and manage. Although the people in this study have experienced profound bodily change, this damage has disturbed, but not destroyed, their embodied selves. These people still inhabit and possess their bodies; their bodies are still resources with which they may explore new possibilities and opportunities of re-embodiment. Although it is not hard to see that such conditions may initially be perceived as a tragedy, the catastrophe may be the catalyst for new ways of using and thinking about the body.

It seems paradoxical that loss of bodily control may precipitate a lessening of social control. No longer mediated through the predictabilities of socialised learning and understanding, the body is experienced in a new and immediate form. For many of the informants, the experience of their fragmented body has presented them with an opportunity to reflect on the nature of their embodied selves, often for the first time. The inability to conform to many aspects of conventional bodily presentation and practice and to the expectations of others has, in a sense, 'left people alone with their bodies' (Shilling 1993, p. 167). While the damage may be immense, the disembodiment opens the way for creative re-embodiment. The living bodies of the informants may explore new and exciting possibilities of bodily experience and practice.

Even so, many of the informants strongly expressed the desire to be as much like other people as possible in terms of bodily appearance and activities. Social connectedness and biographical continuity are abiding concerns, and the status quo may always be more appealing than the spectre of confronting an unknown future. Yet achievement of this goal must involve an active process of disattention to the reality of the damage and disruption that have occurred. While it is not hard to understand why some of the informants might choose this strategy in order to facilitate their re-assimilation into the everyday world of work, family, parenting and relationships, in the long run this goal must be seen as a body-denying strategy. The bodily damage remains, it cannot be wished away. Such deception confines bodies to the rigid parameters of conventional social categories and may deepen and perpetuate the disembodiment caused by the injury or the disease. The disaggregation of embodiment—the separation of self and body, the disjunction between 'me' and 'my body' (Scarry 1985, pp. 48–9)—clearly overrides any more pragmatic gains that this strategy may achieve. In presenting a body for others, the men and women may deny the more critical body for self.

Existence in 'risk society' (Beck 1992) involves living with a mind that is open to the positive and negative possibilities of action. Exposure to a variety of ideas, choosing options from a range of possibilities, the constant monitoring of action and feelings are components of the reflexive project of self by which people negotiate a lifestyle and orient themselves to the future (Giddens 1991). Engagement with the risks and dangers of intimacy exposes bodies to 'contingent happenings' (Giddens 1991, p. 28). Confronting old expectations about the body, and learning to accept that this leaky, unreliable and often troublesome body not only is *my* body, but is a body that is capable of being loved by others, has been a powerful component of re-embodiment for many of the informants. Although assumptions and expectations embedded in conventional gender relations may impede the processes of re-embodiment in these critical areas, it is clear that intimacy is the means by which new bodily pleasures and experiences are discovered, and the embodied self is revitalised.

This study has involved the work of many scholars. The contributions of Berger and Luckman, Bourdieu, Connell, Elias, Foucault, Frank and Goffman to the development of a sociology of the body have been acknowledged in chapter 1, and each has played a role in this study. In drawing on the narratives of people's experiences of bodily disruption and re-embodiment, this study engages with the work of Frank (1991a), Kleinman (1988), Murphy (1987), Plummer (1995), Sacks (1976; 1981; 1984) and Scarry (1985). Plummer's 'personal experience narratives of the intimate' (1995, p. 19), and Scarry's analysis of human suffering, are concerned with the role stories play in social and political change. It is not hard to discern a connection with Giddens (1991) in Plummer's contention that 'the stories we tell of our lives are deeply implicated in moral and political change' (1995, p. 144), but it is the discursive power of language about the body that is central to the work of these writers, not the lived body.

While this study is also concerned with remaking social and political worlds, the project of reconstitution occurs not so much through the discursive reconstruction of language as through the disruptive, ambiguous, reflective and creative possibilities of embodiment. The frailty and vulnerability of the body lie at the heart of this study. Intrinsic to this state is its potential for either enablement and facilitation, or constraint and restriction. The body repeatedly reasserts the fact of its own 'existence, presence, aliveness, realness' (Scarry 1985, p. 193). It is the body that feels, the body that experiences pain and pleasure, and the body that expresses its concerns. This must be seen not as a reversion to the mind–body dualism that has dominated social thought, but rather as a perspective that transcends one-sided, polarised positions to embrace integration and diverse possibilities. The informants have reconstituted their self-identities in terms of rational choices and strategies, but it is the experiences of their frail and damaged bodies that have initiated and directed the body project. Following Merleau-Ponty (1962, pp. 198–9), this study makes the integration of body and mind the framework for an exploration of embodiment.

It is clear that this study cannot be contained wholly within a phenomenological perspective, but nor is a constructionist argument sufficient to understand the processes involved in the reconstitution of the body after severe crisis. There are compelling reasons for viewing the body from both perspectives: as a lived body in the phenomenological tradition and, simultaneously, as a social construction in terms of more recent anti-foundationalist theory. While acknowledging the validity of each position, this study has demonstrated the importance of the integration of these perspectives in order to understand the body in society. In arriving at this position through the exploration of empirical data in this study, I am aligning myself with Turner (1992), Shilling (1993), Lupton (1994), and others who have argued the case for synthesis and integration of the dual positions in sociology. While one must be mindful of the accusation of 'epistemological pragmatism' (Turner 1992, p. 61) that may be associated with such a stance, it is undeniable that although the body is constantly penetrated by the social in the contemporary world, the fragmented, frail, damaged, leaking bodies of the informants in this study have engaged in novel acts of re-embodiment.

DEFINING EMBODIMENT IN A WORLD OF HIGH TECHNOLOGY

Remaking the body takes on new meaning at this late stage of the twentieth century. While the informants in this study have remade their bodies in a variety of creative ways, the rapid development of technology in recent years presents a prospect of hitherto unimaginable possibilities. Reaching far beyond the expectations of simple bodily repair, technology offers the potential to extend the functions and activities of the body, to supplement inadequate performance, to enhance endurance and to heighten experience and sensation.

In the past the organic body and technology have been seen to occupy distinct and incompatible domains. Yet the post-human body has long been the stuff of science fiction. Fascination or horror were evoked by the vision of a monster fashioned of human flesh and techno-parts, alien to our experience and beyond our control. The possibility that our bodies could be taken over by technology and controlled against our will fed our worst fears, and epitomised the terror that lay at the heart of early science fiction.

But technology has not always been constructed as evil: it has been presented in other ways. Joyful advertisements for electric vacuum cleaners and other domestic technology in the fifties promised release from household drudgery. Lee Majors acting in the television series the *Six Million Dollar Man*, was part-human flesh, part-technical system, yet he was the good guy, the hero, the saviour of all. Like people, technology can be good or bad: it can evoke reactions of terror, or people may respond with fascination and enthusiasm to the prospects it offers.

Yet we seldom stop to consider the extent of our everyday reliance on technology. While we have gradually accommodated ourselves to accept a range of pharmacological and surgical interventions to remedy problems in sick or disordered bodies, we are now faced with techniques that can extend the capabilities of bodies far beyond the parameters of what we have assumed was normal. Pushed beyond what we understood as their mandate for bodily rehabilitation or cure, such techniques point to an unimaginable future for the body of unlimited opportunity for choice and reconstruction.

What, then, does embodiment mean in the high-tech world we inhabit in the last years of the twentieth century? Haraway claims that we no longer have a choice to live outside of, or not be shaped by, the technological world and its implications (Haraway 1995, p. xix). '[We] are all chimeras, theorized and fabricated hybrids of machine and organism; in short, we are cyborgs' (Haraway 1991, p. 150). Machines are indissociable human extensions (Haraway 1995, p. xvii). Haraway draws on Douglas's explorations (1966; 1973) of bodily boundaries and social order to explain the anxiety that leaking bodies and social disruption provoke (1991, p. 173). Clearly, the notion of the human organism as a distinct and bounded category can no longer be sustained. Both the organism and society have been thoroughly infiltrated by technology, and both the organism and society are disordered. To think otherwise is to indulge in naive, back-to-nature mysticism (Haraway 1995, p. xvii). But we should not be so alarmed by the blurring of these boundaries. On the contrary, many scholars (Balsamo 1996; Dery 1996; Featherstone & Burrows 1995; Gray 1995; Haraway 1991, 1995; Law 1991; Wajcman 1991) rejoice in the opportunities presented by dismantling the rigid categories of the past. By devolving the power invested in old, discriminatory dualisms, creative new fusions point to a much more optimistic future.

While the word cyborg may for some people evoke an image of

the metal-fleshed warriors of science fiction, cyborgs will be critical to embodiment in the new millennium. Indeed some writers claim that cyborgs represent a fundamentally new stage of human history: a new world order (Gray et al. 1995, p. 6; Haraway 1991, 1995). Although we may be unfamiliar with the word in our everyday lives, we already live in a 'cyborg society' (Gray et al. 1995, p. 3). While a robot is simply a machine, a cyborg is the 'melding of the organic and the machinic' (Gray et al. 1995, p. 2). Machines may be intimately linked and interfaced with humans in almost every aspect of our lives. Artificial organ transplants, pacemakers, prosthetic limbs and breasts, stomas, grafts have become commonplace in clinical medicine: some writers claim that anyone immunised to resist disease or who takes drugs to think, behave or feel better is also technically a cyborg (Gray et al. 1995, p. 2). Put into a perspective of common practice, the cyborg takes on a much less sinister meaning.

It would be wrong, however, to suggest that a cyborg is simply an addition or modification of regular bodily function to increase efficiency or to make a task easier. By weaving together the organic and the technical, cyborgs breach the boundaries between previously incompatible universes. Former distinctions of human–tool, human–machine, organic–inorganic, living–dead can no longer be sustained. Technological innovation thus challenges the coherence of the human body as a discrete organic unity (Clough 1997).

Despite utopian optimism for its limitless and desired possibilities, technology may also present us with a much less positive prospect. While serving the body, technology may also have the potential to supplant the frail, unreliable, leaky body. Technology may be more efficient, less unreliable and less vulnerable than the body. While technology may be the means to make bodies durable in an era of escalating global risk, the predictability, endurance and strength that are created may be at the cost of the integrity of the body. The body may be vulnerable to penetration by others, technology may threaten to engulf the self. In the quest for perfectibility, technology may transcend the body as we know it. We must consider the possibility of a post-human body.

Just as we should reflect upon the source of some people's resistance to cyborgs, we should also reflect upon the implications of embracing them. Optimism for the fluid and diverse possibilities of cyborgs should not blind us to the constraints and conditions that may be operating to impede this vision. The expansive vista wherein everything seems possible may be compromised by the 'realities' which postmodernists may choose not to see. Technology is not born innocent, nor is it neutral. Multinational interests compete for territory in a global world, and retain their power to appropriate new forms and pathways. Although cyberspace offers scope for revisionary possibilities, it seems that the reproduction of gendered binary oppositions is the more likely occurrence (Balsamo 1994, 1996; Wajcman 1991). Rather than embracing the anarchy of freedom, the technologies of virtual reality may retreat to the security of old rules.

It is not hard to imagine that cyberculture may present as an irresistible opportunity to escape our history and our mortality (Dery 1996, p. 10). Transcending both the inevitable decay of the individual body and the social, political, economic and ecological problems that we have created is a seductive promise. Deliverance and escape, however, are seldom simple solutions. By wresting the body from traditional and theological ways of thought, revolutionary science introduced new and secular definitions of the world; but in the process it provided the justification for a whole new range of social discriminations. The expectation that postindustrial technologies would free us from onerous aspects of work has not been realised. The promise of leisure and more time for oneself has quickly turned into a more suffocating form of workplace conscription through laptop computers, modems, video conferences, mobile phones, pagers and a range of other surveillance devices. While the lure of a flexible workplace seems irresistible for workers used to the constraints of the office blocks and industrial spaces of capitalism, privacy and a life of one's own are costly sacrifices. Even the political task of expropriating technology from its 'traditional owners' so that it may be 'collectively imagined by everyone who will one day inhabit it' (Dery 1996, p. 14) seems compromised by poor evidence of empowerment or adjustment of society to the full impact of technology. It seems clear that the engine of liberation may also be an instrument of repression (Dery 1996, p. 15).

In the past, virtue, albeit limited, was afforded those people who bravely accepted the limitations of their bodies, despite the social costs. This dispensation has all but disappeared in an era in which endless possibilities for bodily manipulation exist. If one can choose to alter one's body to reflect particular attitudes, one must accept blame for failing to act in accordance with broad social ideas about proper behaviour, presentation and practice. We can be other than that which we are.

In his famous soliloquy Shakespeare ponders the moral implications of stoicism in the face of the vicissitudes of the body and one's lot in life (*Hamlet*, act 3, scene 1). 'Whether 'tis nobler in the mind to suffer/ The slings and arrows of outrageous fortune,/ Or to take arms against a sea of troubles/ And by opposing end them?' But will death, or cyberspace, '[. . .] end/ The heart-ache and the thousand natural shocks/ That flesh is heir to [. . .]'? Although situated in the domain of sixteenth-century Elizabethan literature, not the

future-present world of cyborgology (Gray et al. 1995, p. 1), Shakespeare's words may serve as a premonition for the project of remaking
bodies in the new millennium as he writes, '[. . .] what dreams
may come/ When we have shuffled off this mortal coil,/ Must give
us pause [. . .].'

And pause is what we must do. For the people in this study, for
us all, apocalyptic dreams of post-human transcendence must be
tempered by more pedestrian strategies for survival. There is no
doubt that we live in risk society (Beck 1992) and that the body is
unstable and unreliable. It is also irrefutable that we inhabit technoculture. Technology is not an aspect of the distant future, it is the
all-encompassing here and now. Embodiment, disembodiment and
re-embodiment occur in this domain. We must acknowledge, as
Haraway does, that 'The machine is not an *it* to be animated,
worshipped, and dominated. The machine is us, our processes, an
aspect of our embodiment' (1991, p. 180). The informants in this
study have demonstrated the enormous resilience and durability of
human embodiment and the power to resist aspects of prevailing
social categories. Their stories are evidence of their ability to re-
imagine and relive their frail and damaged bodies. While no escape,
technology does promise a spectrum of possibilities. In recon-
ceptualising technology as part of our embodiment, rather than as
the enemy, *we* and *it* cease to exist. The synthesis need not be fraught
or fearful. Technology will not disenfranchise the body, '[. . .] the
cyborg is our flesh too [. . .]' (Haraway 1995, p. xvii). The
reassertion of human agency in techno-embodiment promises an
optimistic and creative future. As Haraway says, 'We can be responsible for machines; *they* do not dominate or threaten us. We are
responsible for boundaries; we are they' (1991, p. 180). The liaison
is the promise of the new century.

The possibility of emancipation from the rigid categories of the
past presents men and women with disabilities, indeed all men and
women, with the freedom to experiment with expansive new forms
of bodily expression. Although disability may retain elements of
personal tragedy because of its disjunction with former attachments
and pleasures, technoculture may offer a multitude of opportunities
to free the body from the coercive constraints of the past. These
damaged and fragmented bodies not only epitomise the postmodern-
ist idea of a non-unified body, they are also bodies operating within
a 'cyborg society' (Gray et al. 1995, p. 3). Moreover, people with
disabilities have the potential to be amongst the major beneficiaries
of the technological revolution. Virtual reality sport, for example,
will encourage more inclusive participation: in bypassing the key-
board, a voice-activated computer will connect people in new and
exciting ways. New approaches to rehabilitation will engage people

with disabilities in creative liaisons with others and with technologies as they work on their bodies; these approaches will not leave 'people alone with their bodies' (Shilling 1993, p. 167), but will situate rehabilitation within the broad and expansive ambit of technoculture. Although the context is replete with risk and danger, this study has clearly demonstrated that the embodied actor is an active and creative participant in the process of re-embodiment, now, and in the future.

The millennium presents different opportunities, and a new challenge to dichotomous thought. The disruption and synthesis of the categories 'body' and 'technology' point to more expansive sociologies, redefine embodiment and offer the hope of greater human satisfaction and happiness. The future raises even more profound questions about the body. No longer knowable in terms of old certainties and constraints, the body may be even more elusive in the new millennium. This book ends with the question with which it began: what is the body?

Bibliography

Abdilla, J. 1992 'Good Sense On Sexuality Under Threat' *Link Disability Journal* September/October

ACROD 1988 *Menstruation Aids and Management for Australian Women with Disabilities* Australian Council for the Rehabilitation of the Disabled, ACT, September

Albrecht, G. 1992 *The Disability Business: Rehabilitation in America* Sage Publications, California

Balsamo, A. 1994 'The Body and Technology' Lecture given at University of South Australia, Adelaide, 20 July

——1996 *Technologies of the Gendered Body: Reading Cyborg Women* Duke University Press, USA

Baum, F. 1993 'Deconstructing the Qualitative-Quantitative Divide in Health Research' *Annual Review of the Health Sciences* vol. 3, Centre for the Study of the Body and Society, Geelong, pp. 6–18

Beck, U. 1992 *Risk Society: Towards a New Modernity* Sage, London

Becker, E. 1978 *Female Sexuality Following Spinal Cord Injury* Accent Special Publications, Illinois

Berger, J. 1972 *Ways of Seeing* Penguin, Great Britain

Berger, P. 1990 [1967] *The Sacred Canopy: Elements of a Sociological Theory of Religion* Anchor Books, New York

Berger, P. and Luckman, T. 1966 *The Social Construction of Reality* Doubleday, Garden City, New York

Blumer, M. 1982 *The Use of Social Research* George Allen & Unwin, Sydney

Bogle, J. and Shaul, S. 1981 'Body Image and the Woman with a Disability' in D. Bullard and S. Knight eds *Sexuality and Physical Disability, Personal Perspectives* The C.V. Mosby Company, St Louis

Bourdieu, P. 1978 'Sport and Social Class' *Social Science Information* vol. 17, no. 6, Sage, London and Beverly Hills, pp. 819–40

186

——1984 *Distinction: a Social Critique of the Judgement of Taste* Routledge and Kegan Paul, London

——1988 'Program for a Sociology of Sport' *Sociology of Sport Journal* vol. 5, pp. 153–61

Bowe, M. 1987 'A Woman's Choice? The IVF Option' *Arena* vol. 79, Arena Printing Group, Melbourne, pp. 146–55

Braithwaite, V. 1990 *Bound to Care* Allen & Unwin, Australia

Breckenridge, J. and Carmody, M. eds 1992 *Crimes of Violence. Australian Responses to Rape and Child Sexual Assault* Allen & Unwin, Sydney

Bromley, I. 1976 *Tetraplegia and Paraplegia* Churchill Livingstone, Edinburgh

Browne, S., Connors, D. and Stern, N. eds 1985 *With the Power of Each Breath: A Disabled Women's Anthology* Cleis Press, Pittsburgh

Bryman, A. 1984 'The Debate about Quantitative and Qualitative Research: A Question of Method or Epistemology?' *British Journal of Sociology* vol. 35, no. 1, pp. 75–93

Bryson, L. 1987 'Sport and the Maintenance of Masculine Hegemony' *Women's Studies International Forum* vol. 10, no. 4, pp. 349–60

Bullard, D. and Knight, S. eds 1981 *Sexuality and Physical Disability, Personal Perspectives* The C.V. Mosby Company, St Louis

Bury, M. 1986 'Social Constructionism and the Development of Medical Sociology' *Sociology of Health and Illness* vol. 8, pp. 137–69

Butler, J. 1990 *Gender Trouble: Feminism and the Subversion of Identity* Routledge, Great Britain

Campling, J. 1981 *Images of Ourselves: Women with Disabilities Talking* Routledge and Kegan Paul, London

Cass, B. 1987 'The Family' in S. Encel and M. Berry eds 1987 *Selected Readings in Australian Society* Longman Cheshire, Melbourne, ch. 5

Clarke, A. and Clarke, J. 1982 ' "Highlights and Action Replays"—Ideology, Sport and the Media' in J. Hargreaves ed. *Sport, Culture and Ideology* Routledge and Kegan Paul Ltd, London

Clough, R. 1997 'Sexed Cyborgs? please tick appropriate box. M □ F □ Other □ ' *Social Alternatives* vol. 16, no. 1, January

Cockburn, C. 1990 'Men's Power in Organisations, Equal Opportunities Intervenes' in J. Hearn and D. Morgan eds *Men, Masculinities and Social Theory* Unwin Hyman Ltd, London, pp. 72–93

Cohen, L. and Manion, L. 1989 *Research Methods in Education* 3rd edn, Routledge, London

Colquhoun, D. 1993 'Is There Life in Health Education After Biomedical Research? A Personal Account' *Annual Review of the Health Sciences* vol. 3, Centre for the Study of the Body and Society, Geelong, pp. 60–75

Connell, R. 1983 'Men's Bodies' *Australian Society* vol. 2, no. 9, October

——1987 *Gender and Power: Society, the Person and Sexual Politics* Allen & Unwin, Sydney

Connell, R. and Dowsett, G. eds 1992 *Rethinking Sex. Social Theory and Sexuality Research* Melbourne University Press, Melbourne

Coward, R. 1984 *Female Desire: Women's Sexuality Today* Paladin, London

Cranny-Francis, A. 1992 *Engendered Fictions: Analysing Gender in the*

Production and Reception of Texts New South Wales University Press, Sydney

Daly, J. and Willis, E. 1990 *The Social Sciences and Health Research* The Report of a Workshop on the Contribution of the Social Sciences to Health Research, Public Health Association, Ballarat

Davis, A. 1987 'Women with Disabilities: Abortion and Liberation' *Disability, Handicap and Society* vol. 2, no. 3, pp. 275–84

Davis, A. and George, J. 1993 *States of Health: Health and Illness in Australia* HarperEducational Australia, Sydney

Davis, F. 1963 *Passage Through Crisis*, Bobbs Merrill Co Inc, Indianapolis

Deegan, M. 1985 'Multiple Minority Groups: A Case Study of Physically Disabled Women' in M. Deegan and N. Brooks eds 1985 *Women and Disability* Transaction Books, New Jersey, ch. 4

Deegan, M. and Brooks, N. eds 1985 *Women and Disability. The Double Handicap* Transaction Books, New Jersey

Deem, R. 1987 'The Politics of Women's Leisure' in J. Horne, D. Jary and A. Tomlinson eds *Sport, Leisure and Social Relations* Routledge and Kegan Paul Ltd, London

Dery, M. 1996 *Escape Velocity: Cyberculture at the End of the Century* Hodder & Stoughton, Great Britain

Douglas, M. 1966 *Purity and Danger: An Analysis of the Concepts of Pollution and Taboo* Routledge and Kegan Paul, Great Britain

——1973 *Natural Symbols: Explorations in Cosmology* Penguin Books, Harmondsworth

Dovey, K. and Gaffram, J. 1987 *The Experience of Disability* Victoria College Press, Victoria

Doyal, L. 1979 *The Political Economy of Health* Pluto Press, London

Durkheim, E. 1951 *Suicide: A Study in Sociology* The Free Press, New York

Edgar, D. 1980 *Introduction to Australian Society* Prentice-Hall, Sydney

Elias, N. 1978 *The Civilizing Process: the History of Manners* Basil Blackwell, Oxford

——1991 *The Symbol Theory* Sage, London

Elias, N. and Dunning, E. 1986 *Quest for Excitement: Sport and Leisure in the Civilising Process* Basil Blackwell, Oxford

Emberley, J. 1988 'The Fashion Apparatus and the Deconstruction of Postmodern Subjectivity' in A. Kroker and M. Kroker eds *Body Invaders. Sexuality and the Postmodern Condition* Macmillan Educational Ltd, Hampshire

Emerson, J. 1973 'Behaviour in Private Places: Sustaining Definitions of Reality in Gynaecological Examinations' in K. Thompson and D. Salamon eds *People and Organisations* The Open University, London

Falk, P. 1994 *The Consuming Body* Sage, London

Featherstone, M. 1987 'The Body in Consumer Culture' *Theory, Culture and Society* vol. 1, no. 2, pp. 18–33

——1991 *Consumer Culture and Postmodernism* Sage, London

Featherstone, M. and Burrows, R. eds 1995 *Cyberspace/Cyberbodies/Cyberpunk. Cultures of Technological Embodiment* Sage Publications Ltd, London

Featherstone, M. and Hepworth, M. 1991 'The Mask of Ageing and the

Postmodern Life Course' in M. Featherstone, M. Hepworth and B. Turner eds *The Body, Social Process and Cultural Theory* Sage, London

Featherstone, M., Hepworth, M. and Turner, B. eds 1991 *The Body, Social Process and Cultural Theory* Sage, London

Finch, J. 1984 'It's Great to Have Someone to Talk to: The Ethics and Politics of Interviewing Women' in C. Bell and H. Roberts eds *Social Researching* Routledge and Kegan Paul, London

Fine, M. and Asch, A. eds 1988 *Women with Disabilities: Essays in Psychology, Culture and Politics* Temple University Press, Philadelphia

Finger, A. 1985 'Claiming All Of Our Bodies: Reproductive Rights and Disability' in S. Browne, D. Connors and N. Stern eds *With the Power of Each Breath. A Disabled Women's Anthology* Cleis Press, Pittsburgh

Fishwick, M. 1981 'Sexuality and Attendant Care' *Sexuality and Physical Disability, Personal Perspectives* The C.V. Mosby Company, St Louis

Foucault, M. 1979 *Discipline and Punish: The Birth of the Prison* Penguin, Harmondsworth

——1981 *The History of Sexuality: Volume One: an Introduction* Penguin, Harmondsworth

Frank, A. 1990 'Bringing Bodies Back in: A Decade Review' *Theory, Culture and Society* vol. 7, pp. 131–62

——1991a *At the Will of the Body, Reflections on Illness* Houghton Mifflin Company, Boston

——1991b 'For a Sociology of the Body: An Analytical Review' in M. Featherstone, M. Hepworth and B. Turner eds *The Body, Social Process and Cultural Theory* Sage, London

Friedson, E. ed. 1963 *The Hospital in Modern Society* The Free Press of Glencoe, USA

——1970a *Profession of Medicine: A Study of the Sociology of Applied Knowledge* Harper and Row, New York

——1970b *Professional Dominance* Atherton, New York

——1976 *Doctoring Together: A Study of Professional Social Control* Elsevier, Amsterdam and New York

Game, A. 1991 *Undoing the Social: Towards a Deconstructive Sociology* Open University Press, Buckingham

Game, A. and Pringle, R. 1979 'Sexuality and the Suburban Dream' *Australian and New Zealand Journal of Sociology* vol. 15, no. 2, pp. 4–15

Gehlen, A. 1988 *Man. His Nature and Place in the World* trans. C. McMillan and K. Pillemer, Columbia University Press, New York

Giddens, A. 1976 *New Rules of Sociological Method* Hutchinson, London

——1990 *The Consequences of Modernity* Polity Press, Cambridge

——1991 *Modernity and Self-identity: Self and Society in the Late Modern Age* Polity Press, Cambridge

——1992 *The Transformation of Intimacy. Sexuality, Love and Eroticism in Modern Societies* Polity Press, Oxford

Gilbert, P. and Taylor, S. 1991 *Fashioning the Feminine. Girls, Popular Culture and Schooling* Allen & Unwin, Sydney

Gilroy, S. 1989 'The EmBody-ment of Power: Gender and Physical Activity' *Leisure Studies* vol. 8, pp. 163–71

Glaser, B. and Strauss, A. 1965 *Awareness of Dying* Aldine Publishing Co, Chicago

Goffman, E. 1959 *The Presentation of Self in Everyday Life* Doubleday Books, Garden City, New York

——1963 *Behaviour in Public Places: Notes on the Social Organisation of Gatherings* The Free Press, New York

——1964 *Stigma, Notes on the Management of Spoiled Identity* Pelican Books, Harmondsworth

——1967 *Interactional Ritual, Essays in Face-to-Face Behaviour* Aldine, Chicago

——1968 *Asylums* Penguin Books, Middlesex

Gray, C. ed. 1995 *The Cyborg Handbook* Routledge, New York & London

Gray, C., Mentor, S. and Figueroa-Sarriera, H. 1995 'Cyborgology. Constructing the Knowledge of Cybernetic Organisms' in C. Gray ed. 1995 *The Cyborg Handbook* Routledge, New York and London

Graydon, J. 1983 ' "But it's More Than a Game. It's an Institution" Feminist Perspectives on Sport' *Feminist Review* vol. 13, February, pp. 5–16

Greer, G. 1970 *The Female Eunuch* Paladin, London

——1984 *Sex and Destiny: The Politics of Human Fertility* Secker and Warburg, London

Griffin, C., Hobson, D., MacIntosh, S. and McCabe, T. 1982 'Women and Leisure' in J. Hargreaves ed. *Sport, Culture and Ideology* Routledge and Kegan Paul Ltd, London

Griffiths, P. 1992 'Second Olympics a Phenomenal Success' *Link Disability Journal* November, p. 25

Gunew, S. 1987 'Male Sexuality: Feminist Interpretations' *Australian Feminist Studies* no. 5, Summer, pp. 71–85

Guttman, L. 1967 'History of the National Spinal Injuries Centre' *Paraplegia* vol. 5, pp. 115–26

——1973 *Spinal Cord Injuries* Blackwell, Oxford

Haraway, D. 1991 *Simians, Cyborgs, and Women: The Reinvention of Nature* Free Association Books, London

——1995 'Cyborgs and Symbionts: Living together in the New World Order' in C. Gray ed. 1995 *The Cyborg Handbook* Routledge, New York and London

Hargreaves, J. 1986 *Sport, Power and Culture: A Social and Historical Analysis of Popular Sports in Britain* St Martin's Press, New York

Hearn, J. 1994 'Research in Men and Masculinities: Some Sociological Issues and Possibilities' *Australian and New Zealand Journal of Sociology* vol. 30, no. 1, April, pp. 47–70

Hearn, J. and Morgan, D. eds 1990 *Men, Masculinities and Social Theory* Unwin Hyman, London

Hetzel, B. and McMichael, T. 1987 *The L.S. Factor: Lifestyle and Health* Penguin, Melbourne

Hevey, D. 1992 *The Creatures Time Forgot: Photography and Disability Imagery* Routledge, London

Hindson, A. and Gidlow, B. 1994 'The Myth of the "Trickle-Down" Effect of Top-Level Sports Involvement: An Olympic Case-Study' Unpublished paper, Department of Parks, Recreation and Tourism, Lincoln University, Canterbury, New Zealand

Honneth, A. and Joas, H. 1988 *Social Action and Human Nature* trans. Raymond Meyer, Cambridge University Press, Cambridge

Hume, J. 1990 'Women With Disabilities: How Far Have We Come?' pamphlet, Copyright Joan Hume, March 1990

Illis, L., Sedgwick, E. and Glanville, H. 1982 *Rehabilitation of the Neurological Patient* Blackwell, London

Inglis, K. 1995 'Big Serve of Double-Faults' The Weekend Review, *The Australian* 28–29 January, p. 6

Jenkins, H. ed. 1982 *The Arden Shakespeare: Hamlet* Methuen, London

Johnston, G. ed. 1976 *The Australian Pocket Oxford Dictionary* Oxford University Press, Melbourne

Jones, G. and Davidson, J. 1988 'How Spinal Cord Paralysis Affects Body Image' in M. Salter ed. *Altered Body Image—The Nurse's Role* John Wiley and Sons Ltd, Guildford

Kaplan, G. and Rogers, L. 1990 'The Definition of Male and Female. Biological Reductionism and the Sanctions of Normality' in S. Gunew ed. *Feminist Knowledge. Critique and Construct* Routledge, London

Kellehear, A. 1993 *The Unobtrusive Researcher: A Guide to Methods* Allen & Unwin, Sydney

Kimmel, M. ed. 1987 *Changing Men: New Directions in Research on Men and Masculinity* Sage Publications, California

Kleinman, A. 1988 *The Illness Narratives: Suffering, Healing, and the Human Condition* Basic Books, USA

Koutroulis, G. 1993 'Memory-Work: A Critique' *Annual Review of the Health Sciences* vol. 3, Centre for the Study of the Body and Society, Geelong, pp. 76–96

Krathwohl, D. 1985 *Social and Behavioural Science Research* Jossey-Bass, San Francisco

Kroker, A. and Kroker, M. eds 1988 *Body Invaders: Sexuality and the Postmodern Condition* Macmillan, London

Laqueur, T. 1990 *Making SEX: Body and Gender from the Greeks to Freud* Harvard University Press, Cambridge, Massachusetts

Latour, B. 1988 'The Politics of Explanation: An Alternative' in S. Woolgar ed. *Knowledge and Reflexivity: New Frontiers in the Sociology of Knowledge* Sage, London

Law, J. ed. 1991 *A Sociology of Monsters: Essays on Power, Technology and Domination* Routledge, London

Lawler, J. 1991 *Behind the Screens: Nursing, Somology, and the Problem of the Body* Churchill Livingstone, Melbourne

Lenskyj, H. 1986 *Out of Bounds: Women, Sport and Sexuality* The Women's Press, Ontario

Lenz, R. and Chaves, B. 1981 'Becoming Active Partners' in D. Bullard and S. Knight eds *Sexuality and Physical Disability: Personal Perspectives* The C.V. Mosby Company, St Louis

Lewis, B. ed. 1986 *No Children By Choice* Penguin Books, Melbourne

Link Disability Journal 1987 'A Woman With A Disability Begins Motherhood', December, pp. 26–7

Lonsdale, S. 1990 *Women and Disability: The Experience of Physical Disability among Women* Macmillan, London

Loudon, B. 1992 'Swimmers Back Equality' *The Advertiser* Wednesday, 25 November, p. 21

Loudon, J. 1977 'On Body Products: Human Excretion as a Social Action' in J. Blacking ed. *The Anthropology of the Body* Academic Press, London

Lupton, D. 1994 *Medicine as Culture. Illness, Disease and the Body in Western Societies* Sage, London

Madison, J. 1994 'Integration Through Teamwork: Gender Issues in Health Care Management' Unpublished paper delivered at Flinders University Nursing Education and Research Fund Conference *Towards the Third Millennium* 25 July

Manning, P. 1992 *Erving Goffman and Modern Sociology* Polity Press, Cambridge

Márquez, G.G. 1988 *Love in the Time of Cholera* trans. E. Grossman, Penguin, Harmondsworth

Martin, E. 1987 *The Woman in the Body: A Cultural Analysis of Reproduction* Open University Press, Milton Keynes

——1993 'Science and the History of the Body: the Immune System as the "Currency" of Health' Paper delivered at the Sex/Gender in Techno-Science Worlds Conference, University of Melbourne, 26 June–1 July

Matthews, J. 1984 *Good and Bad Women: The Historical Construction of Femininity in Twentieth-Century Australia* George Allen & Unwin, Sydney

——1987 'Building the Body Beautiful', *Australian Feminist Studies* vol. 5, Summer

Merleau-Ponty, M. 1962 *The Phenomenology of Perception* Routledge and Kegan Paul, London

Messner, M. 1987 'The Life of a Man's Seasons: Male Identity in the Life Course of the Jock' in M. Kimmel ed. *Changing Men: New Directions in Research on Men and Masculinity* Sage Publications Inc, California

Minichiello, V., Aroni, R., Timewell, E. and Alexander, L. 1990 *In-Depth Interviewing: Researching People* Longman Cheshire, Melbourne

Mishkind, M., Rodin, J., Silberstein, L. and Striegel-Moore, R. 1987 'The Embodiment of Masculinity. Cultural, Psychological and Behavioural Dimensions' in M. Kimmel ed. *Changing Men: New Directions in Research on Men and Masculinity* Sage Publications, California

Moore, T. 1991 *Cry of the Damaged Man—A Personal Journey of Recovery* Picador, Sydney

Morgan, G. and Smircich, L. 1980 'The Case for Qualitative Research' *Academy of Management Review* vol. 5, no. 4, pp. 491–500

Morris, J. ed. 1989 *Able Lives. Women's Experience of Paralysis* The Women's Press Limited, London

Murphy, R. 1987 *The Body Silent* Henry Holt and Company Inc, New York

O'Brien, C. 1992 'A Delightful Gift' *Link Disability Journal* September/October, p. 17

Oakley, A. 1981 *Subject Woman* Fontana, Glasgow

——1986 *From Here to Maternity. Becoming a Mother* Penguin Books, England

Oliver, M. 1990 *The Politics of Disablement* The Macmillan Press, London

Parsons, T. 1951 *The Social System* Routledge and Kegan Paul, London

Patton, M. 1990 *Qualitative Evaluation and Research Methods*, Sage, Newberry Park, California

Plummer, K. 1995 *Telling Sexual Stories. Power, Change and Social Worlds* Routledge, London

Pringle, R. 1983 'Women and Consumer Capitalism' in C. Baldock and B. Cass eds *Women, Social Welfare and the State* Allen & Unwin, Sydney, pp. 85–103

——1988 *Secretaries Talk: Sexuality, Power and Work* Allen & Unwin, Sydney

Roth, J. 1963 *Timetables: Structuring the Passage of Time in Hospital Treatment and Other Careers* Bobbs Merrill Co Inc, Indiana

Rousso, H. 1988 'Daughters with Disabilities: Defective Women or Minority Women?' in M. Fine and A. Asch *Women with Disabilities. Essays in Psychology, Culture, and Politics* Temple University Press, Philadelphia

Rowland, R. 1988 *Woman Herself: A Transdisciplinary Perspective on Women's Identity* Oxford University Press, Melbourne

Sabo, D. and Runfola, R. 1980 *Jock–Sports and Male Identity* Prentice-Hall, New Jersey

Sacks, O. 1976 *Awakenings* Penguin Books, Harmondsworth

——1981 *Migraine, Evolution of a Common Disorder* Pan Books, London

——1984 *A Leg to Stand On* Duckworth, London

Sawchuk, K. 1988 'A Tale of Inscription/Fashion Statements' in A. Kroker and M. Kroker eds *Body Invaders: Sexuality and the Postmodern Condition* Macmillan, Hampshire

Scarry, E. 1985 *The Body in Pain: The Making and Unmaking of the World* Oxford University Press, New York

Schiebinger, L. 1987 'Skeletons in the Closet: The First Illustrations of the Female Skeleton in Eighteenth-Century Anatomy' in C. Gallagher and T. Laqueur eds *The Making of the Modern Body. Sexuality and Society in the Nineteenth Century* University of California, California, pp. 42–83

Schilder, P. 1964 'The image and appearance of the human body' New York, John Wiley cited in B. Turner 1992 Regulating Bodies. Essays in Medical Sociology Routledge, London p. 56

Scraton, S. 1987 'Boys Muscle in Where Angels Fear to Tread—Girls' Subcultures and Physical Activities' in J. Horne, D. Jary and A. Tomlinson eds *Sport, Leisure and Social Relations* Routledge and Kegan Paul, London

Seymour, W. 1989 *Bodily Alterations. An Introduction to a Sociology of the Body for Health Workers* Allen & Unwin, Sydney

Shaul, S., Dowling, P. and Laden, B. 1985 'Like Other Women: Perspectives of Mothers with Physical Disabilities' in M. Deegan and N. Brooks eds *Women and Disability* Transaction Books, New Jersey

Shilling, C. 1993 *The Body and Social Theory* Sage Publications, London

Short, S. 1994 'Towards the Democratisation of Health Research' in C.

Waddell and A. Peterson eds *Just Health. Inequality in Illness, Care and Prevention* Churchill Livingstone, Melbourne

Smith, N. and Smith, H. 1991 *Physical Disability and Handicap. A Social Work Approach* Longman Cheshire, Melbourne

Spence, J. 1986 *Putting Myself in the Picture* Camden Press, London

Steinem, G. 1994 *Moving Beyond Words* Allen & Unwin, Sydney

Stewart, T. 1981 'Sex, Spinal Cord Injury, and Staff Rapport' *Rehabilitation Literature* vol. 42, November/December, pp. 11–12

Strauss, A. 1987 *Qualitative Analysis for Social Scientists* Cambridge University Press, Cambridge

Strauss, A. and Glaser, B. 1975 *Chronic Illness and the Quality of Life* The C.V. Mosby Co, St Louis

Strauss, A. et al. about 1980 'Sentimental Work: A Contribution to the Sociology of Work and Occupation' Undated manuscript, USA

Summers, A. 1975 *Damned Whores and God's Police: The Colonisation of Women in Australia* Penguin, Melbourne

Synnott, A. 1993 *The Body Social: Symbolism, Self and Society* Routledge, London

Theberge, N. 1991 'Reflections on the Body in the Sociology of Sport' *Quest* vol. 43, pp. 123–34.

Trieschmann, R. 1980 *Spinal Cord Injuries* Pergamon Press, New York

Turner, B. 1984 *The Body and Society: Explorations in Social Theory* Basil Blackwell, Oxford

——1987 *Medical Power and Social Knowledge* Sage, London,

——1991 'Recent Developments in the Body' in M. Featherstone, M. Hepworth and B. Turner eds *The Body, Social Process and Cultural Theory* Sage Publications Ltd, London

——1992 *Regulating Bodies. Essays in Medical Sociology* Routledge, London

——1994 'Preface' to P. Falk, *The Consuming Body* Sage, London

Turner, B., Eckermann, L., Colquhoun, D. and Crotty, P. eds 1993 'Methodological Issues in Health Research' *Annual Review of the Health Sciences* vol. 3, Centre for the Study of the Body and Society, Geelong

Wajcman, J. 1991 *Feminism Confronts Technology* Allen & Unwin, Sydney

Wallerstein, J. and Blakeslee, S. 1989 *Second Chances* Bantam, London

White, K. 1994 'Nineteenth Century Medicine, Science and Values' in C. Waddell and A. Peterson eds *Just Health. Inequality in Illness, Care and Prevention* Churchill Livingstone, Melbourne

Whyte, W. 1955 *Street Corner Society* University of Chicago Press, Chicago

Williams, C. 1988 'Patriarchy and Gender: Theory and Methods' in J. Najman and J. Western *A Sociology of Australian Society. Introductory Readings* Macmillan, Melbourne

Willis, P. 1982 'Women in Sport in Ideology' in J. Hargreaves ed. *Sport, Culture and Ideology* Routledge and Kegan Paul Ltd, London

Woolgar, S. and Ashmore, M. 1988 'The Next Step: an Introduction to the Reflexive Project' in S. Woolgar ed. *Knowledge and Reflexivity. New Frontiers in the Sociology of Knowledge* Sage, London

Wynne, A. 1988 'Accounting for Accounts of the Diagnosis of Multiple

Sclerosis' in S. Woolgar ed. *Knowledge and Reflexivity. New Frontiers in the Sociology of Knowledge* Sage, London, pp. 101–22

Zola, I. 1981 *Missing Pieces: A Chronicle of Living with a Disability* Temple University Press, Philadelphia

Index